The Epidural Book

WITHDRAWN

The Epidural Book

A Woman's Guide to Anesthesia for Childbirth

Richard Siegenfeld, M.D.

The Johns Hopkins University Press | Baltimore

Note to the reader: The information in this book should by no means be considered a substitute for the advice of qualified medical professionals. This book describes anesthesia for childbirth *in general*. It was not written about your situation. The services of a competent professional should be obtained whenever medical or other specific advice is needed.

All efforts have been made to ensure the accuracy of the information contained in this book as of the date of publication. The author and the publisher expressly disclaim responsibility for any adverse outcomes arising from the use or application of the information contained herein.

© 2008, 2012 Richard Siegenfeld, M.D.
All rights reserved. Published 2012
Printed in the United States of America on acid-free paper
9 8 7 6 5 4 3 2 1

The Johns Hopkins University Press
2715 North Charles Street
Baltimore, Maryland 21218-4363
www.press.jhu.edu

Library of Congress Cataloging-in-Publication Data

Siegenfeld, Richard.
    The epidural book : a woman's guide to anesthesia for childbirth / Richard Siegenfeld.
        p. cm.
    Includes bibliographical references and index.
    ISBN 978-1-4214-0733-3 (hdbk. : alk. paper) — ISBN 978-1-4214-0734-0 (pbk. : alk. paper)
    — ISBN 978-1-4214-0795-1 (electronic) — ISBN 1-4214-0733-7 (hdbk. : alk. paper) — ISBN
    1-4214-0734-5 (pbk. : alk. paper) — ISBN 1-4214-0795-7 (electronic)
    1. Peridural anesthesia—Popular works. 2. Anesthesia in obstetrics—Popular works. I. Title.
    RD85.P4S54 2013
    617.9'64—dc23   2012012456

A catalog record for this book is available from the British Library.

Illustrations by the author

Special discounts are available for bulk purchases of this book. For more information, please contact Special Sales at 410-516-6936 or specialsales@press.jhu.edu.

The Johns Hopkins University Press uses environmentally friendly book materials, including recycled text paper that is composed of at least 30 percent post-consumer waste, whenever possible.

To my parents
Thank you

Contents

Preface

ARE YOU AFRAID OF experiencing uncontrollable or unrelenting pain during childbirth? Have you heard epidural horror stories from people? Perhaps a friend of a friend experienced an epidural that "didn't work," "took forever to get in," or was painful. Or maybe you've heard of someone whose request for an epidural was even refused?

You may feel better knowing just how well an epidural or a spinal could relieve your pain. Even so, you may still be concerned about the potential effects of an epidural or a spinal on your baby. And what about the potential risks to you? Maybe you have a back problem, scoliosis, or a discreet lower back tattoo. Do you wonder how that may affect your anesthetic options?

Are you concerned about what will happen to you and what your choices are for anesthesia if you have a planned or an

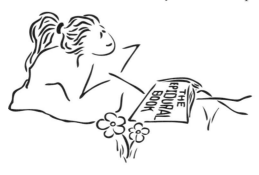

emergency C-section? Are you the type of person who feels better psychologically when you know what is happening to you and what your options are? Do you prefer making informed decisions about your care? Do you appreciate when doctors take the time to explain carefully what they will be doing to you, why, and what to expect in easy-to-understand language, free of medical jargon?

My goal in *The Epidural Book* is to alleviate fear for any woman who anticipates needing an epidural or a spinal for vaginal childbirth. The book does the same for those wondering about anesthesia for a Cesarean section (C-section). I explain procedures in simple ways and address frequently asked questions. This book greatly differs from other labor pain books in its specific focus on anesthesia for the expectant mother: epidurals, spinals, and general anesthesia. It's also purposely lighthearted—to make it more enjoyable to learn what you need to know.

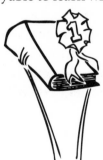

Through many years of performing epidurals for labor and delivery and providing anesthesia for C-sections, I have developed a clear sense of what expectant mothers need to know to feel comfortable with any epidural, spinal, or general anesthetic they may require during childbirth. I have heard nearly every question you can imagine, and I answer the most commonly asked questions and others in the chapters ahead.

Not everyone wants to know everything. Maybe you want to delve into how an epidural is administered but don't want to think about risks, or maybe it's the other way around. This book is designed so that almost any chapter can be read on its own. Information in some chapters is most easily understood by reading another chapter, but I'll let you know when that's the case. Even if you don't read every part carefully, you might want to skim the entire book so that you know what's here.

Epidurals and spinals, from your standpoint, are practically the same. There are only a few subtle differences between them. I initially discuss epidurals in detail. Then, later in the book, I highlight the unique aspects of a spinal. As you read about epidurals, it's fine to assume that you are also reading about spinals, unless I point out specific differences.

The illustrations in this book are not anatomically correct. They are here solely to convey ideas. The opinions in these pages are based on my years of experience as an anesthesiologist. This book does not substitute for individual discussions you should have with your medical caregivers about procedures, their risks, and their benefits.

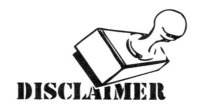

DISCLAIMER

This book may not address a particular condition you have, and it does not cover every problem related to anesthesia. Please appreciate that medical procedures and information evolve over time, and that I do not provide an exhaustive explanation of any procedure. For a more complete explanation, talk with your health care provider.

People are afraid of what they don't understand. I hope this book provides you with a better understanding of what you need to know to make informed decisions without fear.

The Epidural Book

Chapter 1

How Our Thinking and Practice Have Changed

OVER THE PAST 150 years, techniques have evolved to greatly decrease and even eliminate pain during labor. In the

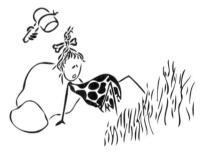

1800s, substances were used, although rarely, to block pain signals traveling along nerves. These substances had names that ended in "-caine" (pronounced "cane"), perhaps the most popular of which was cocaine. Cocaine did not have the negative connotation that it has today. (Modern "-caine" medications that most people have heard of are lidocaine and Novocain.)

In the 1880s, a doctor successfully used cocaine on a patient's eye before eye surgery.[1] (Can you imagine eye surgery without pain-blocking medication?) In the early 1900s, "-caine" medications were injected near nerves responsible for causing pain during childbirth. This procedure was referred to as "regional" anesthesia because it blocked pain signals from only a region, or part, of the body. It was a single injection and lasted only so long.

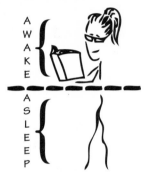

In the 1940s, it was possible to give these medications continuously, but regional anesthesia was still unpopular. At that time, if any medication was used, it was more commonly the kind of medicine that is breathed in. This was referred to as "general" anesthesia. General anesthesia knocks you out: your whole body is affected, not just one part. Only in the past thirty years has the medical community realized how much safer regional anesthesia, like an epidural or a spinal, is than general anesthesia for both the expectant mother and the baby.

Significant improvements have been made in methods for administering regional anesthesia, such as using very thin, long, flexible plastic catheters (tubes) and single use (disposable) supplies. Researchers have conducted thousands of medical studies, and doctors have administered millions of epidurals and spinals, all of which have yielded the modern epidural and spinal available to you.

Despite the general acceptance and proven safety of today's epidurals and spinals, many women still agonize over whether to accept one. For most women, the turmoil revolves around two

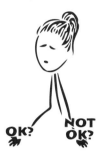

issues. One is that they fear for their own safety and for that of their baby. I hope to ease this fear in the chapters ahead. The other issue is that some women feel as though they are being weak if they opt to have anesthesia when giving birth.

Each of us truly experiences pain differently.[2] If you and your neighbor each set your hands on a hot stove, both of you will be in pain, but your brains will feel the pain differently. Your neighbor may feel it much less than you do. The intensity of pain has nothing to do with who is tougher; it's related to the complex wiring of our internal nervous systems. Also, everyone's

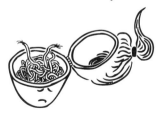

baby is a different size and shape, and is in a different position to pass through the birth canal, which has a shape unique to each woman. No two people are on equal playing fields when it comes to pain.

Try to imagine yourself living back in the mid-1800s and having to undergo a tooth extraction. If you were lucky, you would have been given a couple of shots of bourbon as an anesthetic! If you had the choice today, would you opt against having a shot of Novocain solely to avoid medication, or would you accept a safe, proven technique to get you through having that tooth pulled?

Epidurals and spinals are modern medicine. You would certainly accept an anesthetic today for an operation that, years ago, was performed without anesthesia. Why wouldn't you be just as open to the option of an epidural to block the pain of childbirth?

Finally, I ask you to imagine experiencing anything important in your life, from taking in the beauty of a work by Van Gogh, to filling your studio with the tunes of a rock concert or a piano symphony, to listening to a child whispering in your ear. Would you appreciate them equally with and without pain, or would pain take away from your experience?

As you can tell, I believe that most women don't need to feel all the pain of childbirth when safe and effective procedures like an epidural and a spinal are available. Now let's look at why you'll have pain during childbirth in the first place, and what can be done about it.

Chapter 2

How an Epidural Works

$\mathcal{P}$AIN, ANYWHERE IN YOUR body, starts from a source: your hand touching a hot stove, a bug flying into your eye, an infected appendix. The hand on the hot stove causes a pain signal to travel up a nerve to your brain—which may order your mouth to shout "%$#@!," completely bypassing that filter your parents installed years ago.

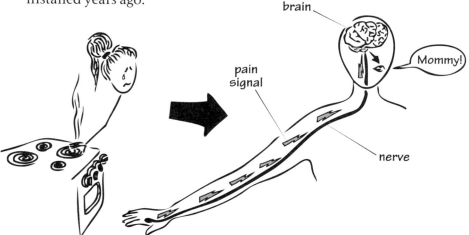

Pain is your defense mechanism to protect you—to tell you to pull your hand away, get the bug out of your eye, or see a doctor about your stomach ache. During childbirth, other than signaling that labor has begun and is progressing, pain is not particularly useful.

Your pain during childbirth will stem from successive contractions of your uterus and, in a vaginal birth, the passage of your baby through your birth canal. Similar to what happens when you touch a hot stove, the pain signal travels along nerves from where it hurts—the uterus and cervix area and the vaginal and rectal area—to your brain.

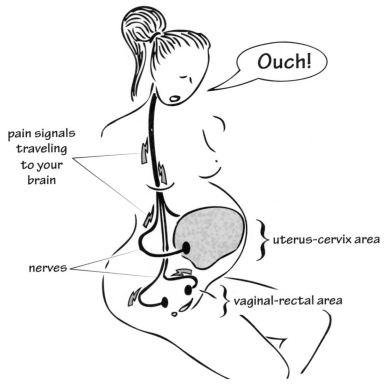

One small but important detail about the nerves that are carrying all those pain signals to your brain is that they must travel through the "epidural space." Imagine each nerve traveling through a sort of two-layer sleeve. The space between the layers is the epidural space. Nerves pass through the epidural

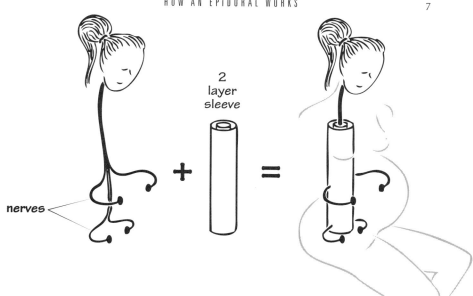

nerves

2
layer
sleeve

space first, before they head up to the brain. The epidural space is where anesthetic medicine is injected to block the pain signals.

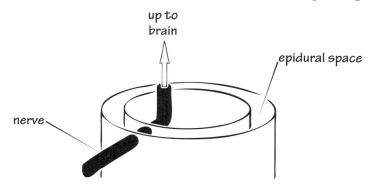

up to
brain

epidural space

nerve

Let's move away from talking about the epidural space for a moment and talk more about pain. If your pain signals can be blocked along their course to your brain at absolutely any point along their path, then voilà, you're pain free. Wouldn't it be great if we could just rub the medicine on your skin, let your skin absorb it, and not disturb anything other than the pain nerves that need to be blocked?

Unfortunately, there is no magic lotion or even a pill to do this. But an epidural is the next best thing. A small catheter (a tiny plastic tube like a miniature hose) can be placed easily in the epidural space, and medicine can be pushed through the catheter to fill the space. After the medicine (the "caine" substance mentioned in chapter 1) is injected, it reaches the nerves

epidural catheter

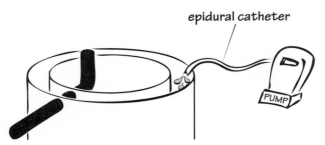

as they pass through the epidural space and blocks the pain signal. Because your brain does not receive these pain signals, you are able to experience labor painlessly.

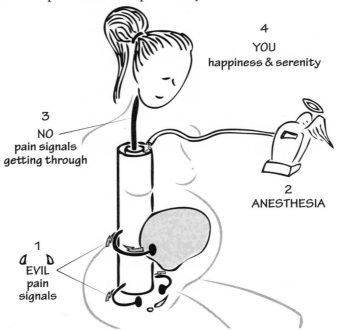

Chapter 3

Where, Who, and When

*I*F YOU DECIDE YOU want an epidural, who decides when you will get it and who will put it in? Ninety percent of the time, these decisions are made for you, either by your obstetrician or by fate. Women usually pick their obstetrician based on advice from family and friends, which is truly a great way to go. But what about your anesthesiologist, the doctor who will be your guardian angel during your labor and delivery?

Most women need only consider the anesthesiologist's ability to place a well-functioning epidural or spinal when it's needed. But anesthesiologists do much more than the important job of addressing pain. If anything goes significantly wrong with your health during labor, delivery, or the days following your delivery, the anesthesiologist may be critical in your care. Can you pick your anesthesiologist? Yes and no, since anesthesiologists come along with the hospital.

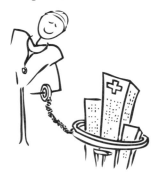

When you choose your obstetrician, you're indirectly choosing a mini-organization too. This organization consists of the hospital your obstetrician is affiliated with and all its personnel, from nurses to anesthesiologists. Having faith in your obstetrician also means having faith in the decisions he or she makes for you, including which hospital you will be going to, and feeling secure that your doctor has confidence in the hospital staff members who will be caring for you.

Nonetheless, it's a great idea to have some clue about the personnel available to you in the labor and delivery unit. By the way, the "obstetric (OB) ward," "labor and delivery," the "birthing section," the "L&D unit," or any combination of these terms all refer to the same thing—the place in the hospital where you will be giving birth to your baby.

You might consider these questions about the hospital and its anesthesiologists. First, are the anesthesiologists in the hospital twenty-four hours a day, seven days a week, and dedicated to just the L&D unit? Or are they not in the hospital at all when the hospital does not have any patients who need their expertise? In some smaller hospitals, with less busy L&D units, anesthesiologists take "call" from home. "Call" means they are literally called to come in only as needed during off-hours, such as at night and on weekends.

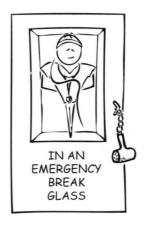

IN AN
EMERGENCY
BREAK
GLASS

Second, do the hospital and the anesthesiology group accept your health insurance? Surprisingly, not all hospitals and anesthesiology groups accept the same insurance that your obstetrician accepts. A phone call to both the hospital and the anesthesia department early in your pregnancy will ward off future surprises to your wallet.

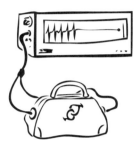

Finally, is the hospital a teaching hospital? Some people don't want doctors-in-training, called interns or residents, learning how to be doctors by caring for *them*. However, some of the best medical care you can receive is at teaching hospitals. Studies have proven this![3] Some hospitals that are not teaching hospitals affiliated with a medical school or medical residency training program still have interns and residents. These hospitals are not formally called teaching hospitals, but they do have visiting student doctors training there under the supervision of seasoned doctors.

Getting answers about the hospital doesn't require doing a ton of homework. Asking your obstetrician these few questions will suffice. He or she will know the hospital and the staff, including the anesthesiologists, very well.

So you're the well-informed expectant mom: you have all your t's crossed and i's dotted. The second coat of paint in the baby's room is just about dry, your hospital bag is packed, and you go into labor. How soon can you get the epidural if you want one?

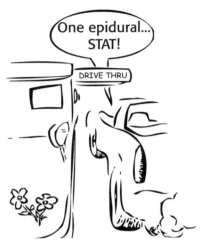

I know women who would vote for epidural service in the hospital's lobby. Of course, in our imperfect world, we have to settle for when the obstetrician gives the okay and after a couple of safety measures are in place. (The safety details are addressed in the next chapter.)

In the past, to get an epidural, your cervix had to be dilated three to five centimeters and your contractions had to be consistent and frequent. The requirements have changed now that modern obstetrics is completely accepting of epidurals. In the United States there are more than 4 million births each year, and a majority of women get epidurals, so if you choose to get one you'll be in good company.

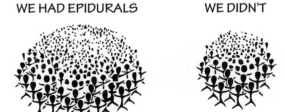

Before authorizing an epidural, today's obstetricians still insist on a couple of things: first, you have to be in labor, and second, your baby must be "comfortable" with the contractions you are having. The baby's comfort is judged by the obstetrician and is based on changes in the baby's heart rate during contractions. Now that definitive studies have demonstrated that epidurals don't prolong dilation or increase the chance for a C-section, you can often receive an epidural earlier in labor than doctors previously allowed.

A few situations may delay or prevent you from getting an epidural or a spinal. Some of these situations can't be addressed until you're in the delivery room, but others can be addressed months before your delivery date. These situations are discussed in chapter 10.

Chapter 4

The Preparation

$\mathcal{T}$HE OBSTETRIC TEAM IS made up of your nurse, your obstetrician, and possibly a resident (physician-in-training) or nurse-practitioner. Once you are in labor and have arrived at the hospital, the team prepares you for labor and delivery. They will admit you to the hospital, which means completing obligatory paperwork. They will ask you a few of the same questions at least three times. This is not because we health care providers don't communicate with one another but because we are all trained to

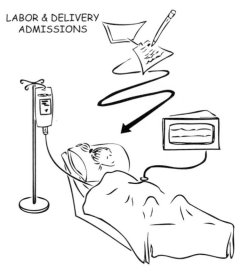

LABOR & DELIVERY
ADMISSIONS

get the story straight from the source: you. Every now and then an important detail is missed by one person only to be discovered by the next. Once you are settled in your birthing room and have changed into a gown, they will do an obstetric exam, start an IV in your arm, and hook you up to a contraction and fetal heart rate (FHR) monitor.

This sounds like a bit much, but an efficient, finely tuned labor and delivery unit can go from "hello" to having you in bed with your hospital PJs on in under twenty minutes if they're in a rush. Saying that you think you see the baby's head reliably moves things along, but I strongly recommend that, instead of exaggerating, you follow a strategy of expedient cooperation and understanding. That way, if another expectant mother actually does see the baby's head, she'll get to jump ahead of you—that's only fair.

Once you're tucked in and the OB team members are satisfied with your contractions and your baby's heart rate, then they can okay you for an epidural (or a spinal), if you want one. Or they

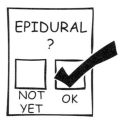

may decide that you're not quite ready yet. In this circumstance, if you are one of those people who would vote for epidural service upon arrival in the hospital lobby, don't panic! In lieu of an epidural, your obstetrician can give you another kind of medication in your IV to help with the pain.

The IV medication does have some downsides: it can make you groggy, it isn't quite as effective as an epidural, and it has a limited duration. Chapter 14 covers alternatives to epidurals and spinals in more detail. Chances are good that if you receive the alternative medication, it means you aren't very far along in labor. The IV medication can easily "bridge" you until you are ready for an epidural.

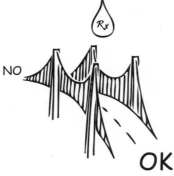

If you are contemplating having some medication to help with pain until you are ready for an epidural, you may want to ask to speak to the anesthesiologist before you receive anything. That way your mind will be clearer, so you can discuss any concerns and ask any questions you have, and you will be able to process the anesthesiologist's answers.

On the other hand, you may want an epidural, be ready for an epidural, and receive an epidural pronto. The nurse will hydrate you by letting a whole bag of IV fluid pour through your IV into you. This step is important because it helps your body

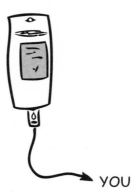

counteract a temporary dip in blood pressure that frequently happens after the epidural or spinal is administered. The IV fluid can take anywhere from five to ten minutes to get into you, depending on how quickly your IV runs. The OB nurse may put a simple device, called a "pressure bag," on the IV fluid bag to literally squeeze the fluid into you faster.

While you're getting hydrated, your nurse is also getting in touch with the anesthesiologist, letting him or her know that you are ready for your epidural.

The anesthesiologist will review your chart, ask you some questions about your medical history, discuss the procedure, and answer any of your questions. If you're a healthy and fairly well-informed expectant mom, all this will take about five to ten

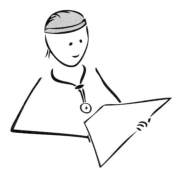

minutes, depending on how complicated your history is, how detailed your questions are, and how detailed an explanation the anesthesiologist provides. A quick word about my colleagues throughout the country and their explanations of procedures and risks: anesthesiologists come in more flavors than ice cream. Some can be a little stingy on the details. To their credit, they are only trying to relieve your pain as quickly as possible. Ideally, after reading this book, you will know a lot about epidurals and spinals and won't need to hope for a very talkative anesthesiologist.

Occasionally, more than one woman needs an epidural at the same time. The person who is ready first usually gets it first. You can sway the odds in your favor by asking to speak to the anesthesiologist *before* you actually want the epidural or are ready for the epidural. You can even talk with the anesthesiologist and decide not to get an epidural at all—no worries. That early chat, combined with the pressure bag on the IV, should nicely speed things along if you suddenly decide you want an epidural.

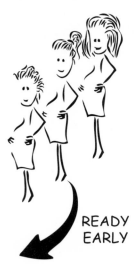

READY
EARLY

There's another benefit of requesting an early anesthesiology visit. Some women have medical conditions that require blood tests be done before an epidural (or a spinal) can be safely administered. The results of the blood tests can't be older than a few hours before the epidural (or spinal) is to be placed. An early visit will allow the anesthesiologist to alert the OB team to obtain a new set of lab tests quickly. Lab tests can take an hour to process, so this early heads up may get you pain relief sooner than if you wait to talk with the anesthesiologist. Situations that require such recent blood tests are discussed in greater detail in chapter 10. My estimate is that such conditions occur in about one in twenty women seeking epidurals.

All right:

> You've selected your hospital and your OB doctor,
> you're in labor,
> you've been admitted to the hospital,
> you've been interviewed,
> you're in your hospital PJs,
> you're fully intravenously hydrated,

and now

> you're dreading the epidural procedure.

Fear not! The next chapter takes you painlessly through the placement of an epidural step by step, to help allay your fears. Knowing how something works can take the anxiety away.

Chapter 5

The Procedure

*T*HE MOST COMMON QUESTIONS women ask me about epidurals relate to how the procedure is administered. I am most often asked:

> Will it hurt?
> What if I get a contraction and suddenly move?
> How fast can it be placed and how fast will it start working?

And

> How long will it last?

Every woman contemplating an epidural has expectations based on what she has heard and what she has read, or even what she has experienced during a previous labor and delivery. It is my personal quest to provide information that makes it possible for every woman to have realistic expectations and a great experience.

As noted earlier, in this book I focus on the epidural procedure. Spinals are similar, with only a couple of exceptions. The subtle differences between epidurals and spinals are addressed in this chapter and in chapter 11.

Although some women fear getting epidurals more than they fear childbirth itself, after receiving an epidural, most women say that the procedure is less uncomfortable than an IV or than even one contraction.

Many women understandably worry about the size of the needle, but needle size ultimately doesn't matter. This is because an initial, truly tiny needle is used to numb the area just before the epidural needle is inserted. That's right: *before*. Most women don't mind this tiny needle. They do, however, feel the numbing medication that is injected through the needle: it stings for five seconds and then starts to work.

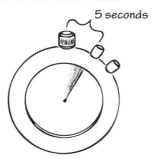

5 seconds

That's really the worst of a typical epidural for most women: a five-second stinging sensation that lasts for a fraction of the duration of one contraction. After those five seconds, you will probably feel a bit of pressure. I can't tell you how many times I've finished administering the epidural only to have the woman tell me that she couldn't believe this was the procedure she'd obsessed over for weeks or months. Patients don't respond as they do because I have magical hands—which, of course, I do!—but because the initial numbing medication is usually the worst part of the whole procedure.

In short, the procedure goes like this. You get into position, cleaning solution is swirled on, you get the numbing medication, and the epidural needle goes through the numb area (and you feel a little bit of pressure). The epidural catheter is threaded into your epidural space (with either no pain or possibly a one-second "hit-your-funny-bone"–like sensation down a leg), the needle is removed, and the catheter is taped to your back. You lie down (but you can't feel the thin catheter), meds are pushed through the catheter, and, finally, you're connected to a pump that continually replenishes the epidural medication until you deliver.

Follow your OB nurse's or anesthesiologist's instructions and you will almost certainly be surprised by how quickly and easily the epidural is done.

Now back to my patients' questions. They ask me

> How will I be positioned during the epidural?
> What if I can't stay still?
> Can the epidural be put in between contractions?
> What happens if I move?
> How do you know you're in the right place and not hitting my nerve, nerves, or spinal cord?
> When will it start to work and how long will it last?
> What if it runs out?
> Will it slow down or speed up labor?
> Can I walk to the bathroom after?
> Will I be able to push at the end?

I am going to answer these questions now, so if you already have enough information about the procedure to your liking, you can skip ahead to chapter 6 at this point. Just as anesthesiologists, obstetricians, and nurses have different personalities, different expectant moms have different personalities. Some will feel that the information already provided in this chapter is way more than enough; they will prefer to leave these other questions unanswered. "Spare me the details, doc!" Alternatively, if you'd like to know the answers to these questions, then please read on.

How will you be positioned during your epidural? We position some women on their side and ask other women to sit up during the epidural. You probably won't be offered a choice. Either way, your OB nurse will help get you into the necessary position.

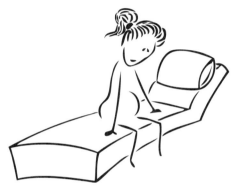

We'll also ask you to try to curl yourself into a little ball. Be prepared for us to use a metaphor or two (or three) to help you understand what exactly you're supposed to do. We might ask you to make your back look like an angry cat, or to push your back out like the letter C, or to wrap around your baby, or to try to make your back like a cooked shrimp, and so on. Good positioning makes your epidural space easily accessible. The easier it is for us to reach your epidural space, the easier it is for you.

Most often, the epidural space is easy to find. Sometimes, however, it is not. When you curl your back like an angry cat, you are spreading open a pathway to make it easier for us to get into the epidural space. We'll press our fingers on your back to help locate the starting points of potential pathways.

Although anesthesiologists are sometimes confused with superheroes (just ask our moms), we don't have x-ray vision. Even if we start at a spot that seems like it would be a wide open pathway and you are doing the world's best cooked shrimp impersonation, the path could still be too small to pass by. If this happens, the anesthesiologist will numb you in a different location and try again. The cost to you: five more seconds of stinging from that numbing medication.

If you're not doing the world's best cooked shrimp impersonation, then you *are* contributing to the problem. Remedy this by pushing your shoulders down and rounding your back out.

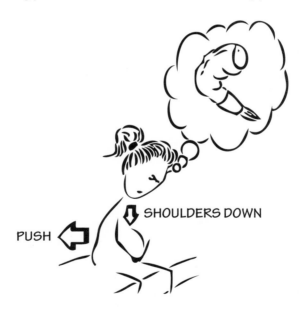

Recall, from chapter 2, that the anesthesiologist's goal is your happiness and serenity. Of course, the epidural medication doesn't pour down from the top, as illustrated in the next figure, to fill your epidural space. The medication enters from the lower

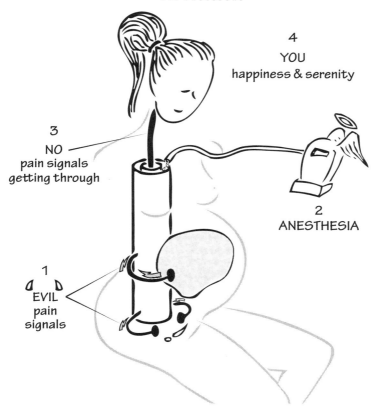

4
YOU
happiness & serenity

3
NO
pain signals
getting through

2
ANESTHESIA

1
EVIL
pain
signals

back, where the epidural is inserted. Once you are in great position, or at least trying as hard as you can, the anesthesiologist will clean off your lower back with a cold cleaning solution and numb the area with that tiny needle. The epidural needle is

numb area

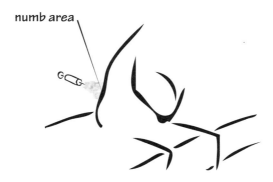

then quickly and gently pushed through this numbed area. You should only feel pressure during this part of the procedure.

We know we're in the epidural space because we feel a change in the syringe attached to the epidural needle. We can easily feel this change. When your anesthesiologist finds your epidural space—and finding it can take as little as 60 seconds—he or she will go ahead and thread the epidural catheter in.

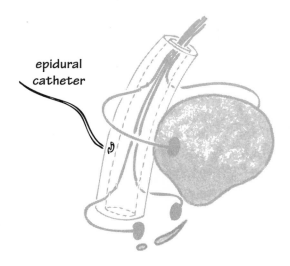

epidural catheter

A quick explanation of your nerves and your spinal cord will help you understand how safe you are. A common misperception is that the epidural (or spinal) is placed *into* a nerve or *into* the spinal cord. Nothing could be further from the truth. The needle, catheter, and medication go into the *compartment* that the nerves pass through.

Your spine is a protective bone structure surrounding your epidural space. Nerves from all over your body, including the ones (illustrated in chapter 2) from the uterus-cervix and vaginal-rectal areas, pass between openings in the spine and then through the epidural space. Then they join as one large bundle and travel up to the brain. This joined bundle of nerves is called the spinal cord. The spinal cord is surrounded by fluid.

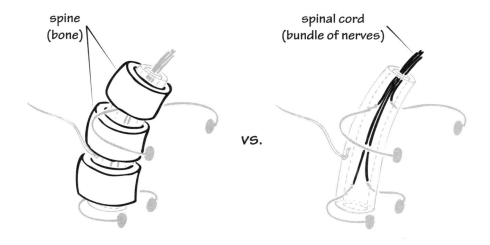

spine
(bone)

spinal cord
(bundle of nerves)

vs.

Bumping into the spine (the bone) with the epidural needle should not matter, and it should not hurt. In fact, you will probably not realize it if your anesthesiologist bumps into the spine. Openings between the bones are the pathways to the epidural (or spinal) compartment he or she is looking for—the pathways mentioned above, in our discussion on getting you into the right position for the procedure.

On the other hand, it is extremely difficult to bump any nerves, especially your spinal cord, with the epidural needle. The spinal cord is deeper than the epidural space. The nerves enter the epidural space from the sides, not from the center—and the needle is placed in the center. Furthermore, if the needle were to enter the space where the spinal cord is, clear fluid would come out the other end of the needle, which is typically quite obvious. The following diagram will give you an idea of what's what:

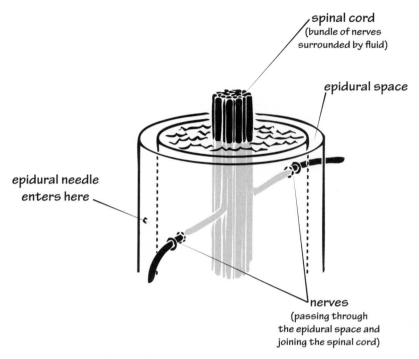

spinal cord
(bundle of nerves
surrounded by fluid)

epidural space

epidural needle
enters here

nerves
(passing through
the epidural space and
joining the spinal cord)

Sometimes the epidural catheter, as it is being threaded, does brush against a nearby nerve, causing a one-second "funnybone"–like sensation down a leg. If this happens and you have not been warned about it, you might think that something has gone terribly wrong. Not so. Although no exact data are available

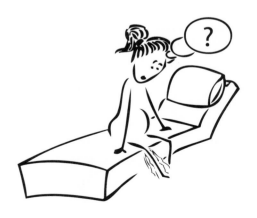

on how often this happens, I would estimate that it occurs in roughly one out of every ten epidurals. Do not be concerned, but do tell the anesthesiologist exactly what you are feeling.

Then the needle is pulled out, and there is no needle left in you. I repeat: THERE IS NO NEEDLE LEFT IN YOU! Only part of the catheter (the tiny tube) is left inside. The rest of the catheter is securely taped to your back. Once the catheter is taped, you get to lie down right on it. It's truly too small to feel. You won't hurt it, and it won't hurt you.

Next, you get a little test medication. Despite our best efforts, the epidural catheter occasionally winds up where we'd rather

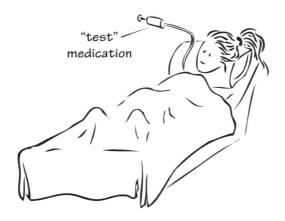

it not be. The epidural space is not infinitely large, and it is not empty. Blood vessels run within it, and it has another side opposite to the spot we enter. If the catheter pokes into a blood vessel or if it pokes through the opposite side, we want to know. The test medication will quickly (usually within two minutes) alert us to a problem, if there is one. If there is a problem, you might suddenly feel dizzy, hear a strange sound like ringing or buzzing, get a funny taste in your mouth (as if you were sucking on a nickel), or feel your legs rapidly becoming extremely numb and weak. *You don't need to remember any of these specific details*, but if you feel different or strange, speak up and let everyone know. The anesthesiologist will be asking how you're feeling anyway and will tell you if what you are experiencing is normal or not.

Once you "pass" this test, the anesthesiologist will give you more medication, which will spread within your epidural space. When the medicine contacts the nerves, any pain signals will be blocked.

The epidural catheter is actually a tiny sterile plastic tube about as thick as a fishing line. The other end—the end that is located outside of you—is connected to a supply of medicine that intermittently or continuously flows through this tube to block the nerves from sensing pain. In most cases, a specially designed pump delivers a fixed amount of medication every few seconds. The medication in the pump is usually a little less concentrated than the initial dose. New medication slowly replaces

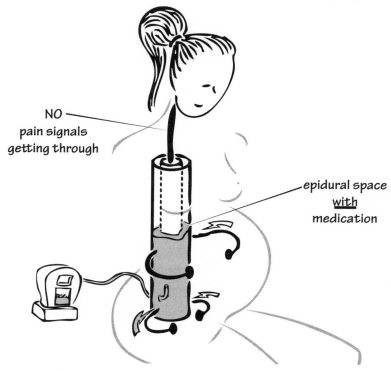

NO
pain signals
getting through

epidural space
with
medication

the medication already in your body so that the effect of the epidural does not wear off.

Even though describing the procedure takes an entire chapter, the epidural can take as little as ten minutes. That's great considering the uncomfortable part is primarily the five seconds of dealing with that initial numbing medication. During the ten minutes of the procedure, however, you will probably have a couple of contractions.

Although a few anesthesiologists suggest that even the slightest movement during the procedure may lead to disaster, this is simply not true. Placing an epidural (or a spinal) is *not* an extremely delicate process. Women who make a small to moderate movement during the procedure slow us down and, in extreme cases, increase their chances of getting a headache afterward. But almost everyone—and that includes you—can stay still enough. Labor contractions can be as frequent as every two minutes; it's unlikely that an epidural could be put in place between contractions that are coming this fast. You'll have a couple of contractions during placement . . . it's okay.

The epidural medication starts to work within five minutes and peaks in ten minutes. Therefore, it'll typically take about fifteen minutes from the moment we start the procedure to the moment you feel relief from pain.

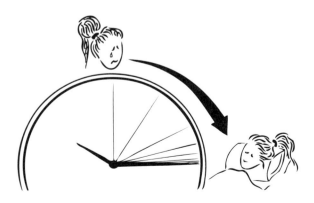

Your legs may feel tingly and a little weak by this time. Because of this, it is not safe for you to be moseying down the hallways to check out the new arrivals. Plan on staying bed-bound for the rest of your labor. Besides, your obstetric team will want your baby's heartbeat and your contractions monitored frequently, and this can only be done from bed. There are obvious impracticalities to this arrangement. Bathroom concerns are addressed either via a bedpan or a urinary catheter. Some hospitals offer "walking" epidurals, which initially don't limit you to your bed as much. These less common epidurals are discussed in chapter 11.

Don't be surprised if one leg or side is more "asleep" than the other. When the epidural catheter is threaded in, it often sways a little to the left or right. Also, no one's back is perfectly symmetrical, and asymmetry can affect the position of the epidural catheter. No one can control these variables, and it does not matter as long as you are comfortable afterward.

The pump or other device that is delivering the epidural medication will be refilled as necessary throughout your labor. Occasionally, obstetricians like to turn down the epidural infusion—the volume of medication a woman is receiving over time—as she nears delivery. Epidurals have been shown to have no effect on the duration of cervical dilation or on whether you get a C-section, but sometimes they extend the duration of pushing at the very end.[4] In some women, epidurals can hamper the ability to push. The average duration of pushing for a woman with an epidural is about twenty minutes longer than for a woman without an epidural. This is why some obstetricians reduce the infusion as the time for delivery comes near. The possibility of increased pushing time will not translate into a higher likelihood of a C-section, as I discuss in more detail in chapter 8.

Some women want to know exactly what medication they are getting. If you are one of them, then here's what you want to know: the usual medication is one of the "-caine" medications, as mentioned in chapter 1 (often bupivacaine or ropivacaine). These "-caine" medications are combined with a small amount of a narcotic (often fentanyl or sufentanyl). The narcotic can make you itch a little bit, particularly around your nose.

Well, that's the perfect epidural, and likely to be exactly what you'll experience. We'll discuss those less common, less than perfect, epidurals in chapter 6. (FYI, we can fix almost anything.)

Chapter 6

The Imperfect Epidural

*O*KAY, YOU'RE DOING GREAT! You got through the procedure, you're thrilled that there really wasn't that much to it, and now you're lying down. Your stomach and legs are feeling warm and tingly, as they should. A few minutes later the pain is gone, though you may still be feeling a little pressure with each contraction. You go to sleep, watch an episode of *Mad Men*, tune into some Japanese flute music: you're in Zen heaven.

Some women who reach this usually blissful point are concerned that their feet aren't as numb as they imagined they'd be.

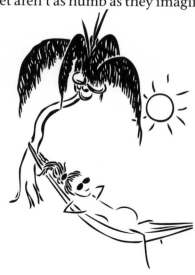

I reassure them that an ideal epidural takes away all the pain while leaving the rest of the senses as intact as possible. Sometimes women reach a Zen-like state, but then, a couple of hours later, they start feeling more and more pressure, even a little pain, say on the left side, with each contraction. If this is you, don't panic. Almost anything is fixable. Let's take a closer look at what's really happening.

Recall from chapter 2 that pain signals travel via nerves from your uterus-cervix area and your vaginal-rectal area to your brain. Also remember that the epidural medication, as it fills the epidural space, blocks these

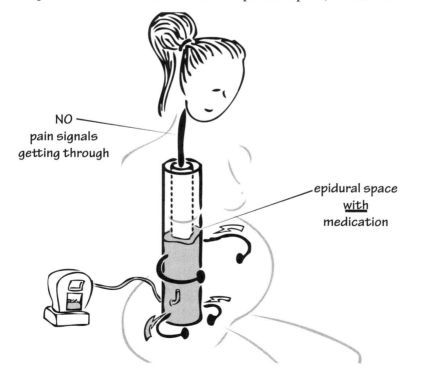

NO
pain signals
getting through

epidural space
with
medication

pain signals. Let's take a closer look at just where the nerves pass through the epidural space. For clarity's sake, I'll rotate the diagram as if you're looking at a person's back. Now I'll expand the view of the important part of the anatomy. (By the way, if

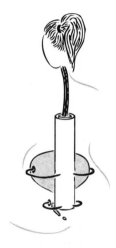

anatomical details are not your thing, you should still continue reading the next few pages. The main ideas are conveyed for anatomy lovers and anatomy haters alike.)

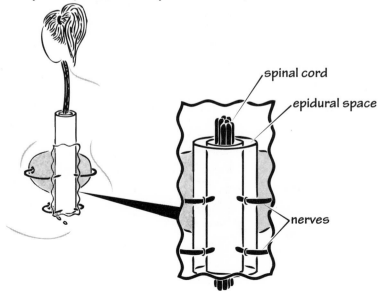

There are two essential bits of information to understand. First, the epidural medication always spreads unevenly within the epidural space. This is likely because the epidural catheter is always located a little more to one side or the other. It really doesn't matter as long as *enough* medication gets to both the left and right sides of your body. Second, when your epidural is first started, the anesthesiologist gives you a good amount of *strong* epidural medication that lasts about sixty to ninety minutes. That medication, as it wears off, is replaced by *weaker* medication pushed through your epidural catheter by a pump every few seconds. The amount given is simply an educated guess of what the average person needs for the average epidural, with small adjustments made depending on your height.

Occasionally the catheter, and therefore the medication, is located just too far to one side. Or you could have a perfectly

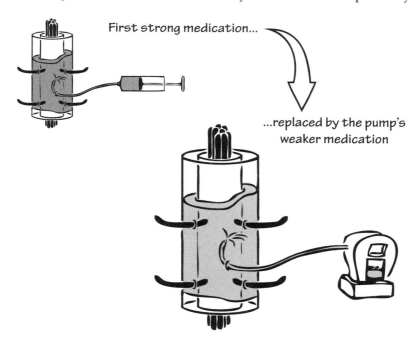

First strong medication...

...replaced by the pump's weaker medication

positioned epidural catheter spreading the medication every-where, but because of your anatomy or physiology, you require a stronger than usual concentration of medication. Either way, the pain signals squeak through.

pain signals
still
getting through

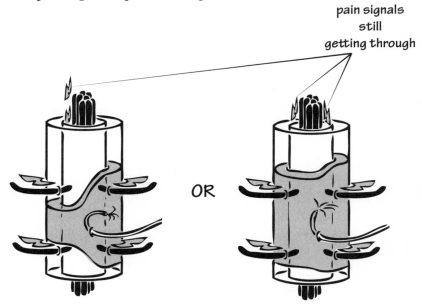

OR

Both of these common problems (too little medication on one side or medication that is too weak) are easily fixed with one solution: an extra dose of strong epidural medication. You may very well need an extra dose or even two or three. These extra doses are sometimes called "boluses," or "top ups."

If this happens to you, at some point you will think that your wonderful epidural is working less wonderfully than it had been. You will express this disappointment to your nurse, who will promptly call the anesthesiology personnel, who, in turn, will likely give the bolus. *The bolus is not only stronger but it also fills up more of your epidural space by sheer volume.* This increases the chances that all your nerves from the uterus-cervix area as well as the vaginal-rectal area will be treated with enough epidural medication.

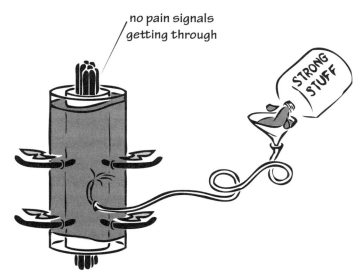

Many women in this situation ask me whether it's okay for them to be getting all this extra medication or why they are not getting the super strong medication all the time. To answer the first question: if the obstetric team believes that your baby is tolerating your contractions well, then there is no problem with your receiving multiple doses of extra epidural medication. If, on the other hand, the team is unsure, you may not be able to receive extra doses just yet. This concern generally has more to do with the temporary dip in your blood pressure than with any bolus. The baby does not directly receive your epidural medication. The medication is placed around your nerves, not into your bloodstream. You'll be happy to know that in no way is your team overdosing you: There is an extremely large difference between the amount we know is too much and what we give women, even with all the additional boluses some women require. In fact, you would be given much less than is needed for a typical C-section.

The answer to the second question has to do with pushing the baby out at the end of labor. Obstetricians sometimes assist deliveries with forceps or a gentle suction device. Some studies have shown that this need is increased with epidurals.[5] As you get closer and closer to full dilation (10 cm) of your cervix, your obstetrician may be more reluctant to give you an extra bolus. The stronger the medication, the more other nerves (besides the pain nerves) are blocked. These other nerves give you muscle strength in your abdomen and legs. They are, fortunately, much less sensitive to medications than the pain nerves are. Your anesthesiologist will usually tweak the strength so that you can be reasonably comfortable and still be able to push your baby out.

Another common situation is for women to feel increasing pressure as they near delivery and to think the epidural is wearing off. This stems from how the medicine spreads within the epidural space. In actuality, the epidural usually winds up closer to your uterus-cervix nerves than to your vaginal-rectal nerves. Also, when you receive boluses, the medication tends to travel upward, toward your head, rather than downward, toward your bottom. Throughout your labor, your uterus and cervix areas will be continually trying to send pain signals to your brain. As your cervix dilates more and more, the baby's head will start to press downward, putting pressure on your vaginal-rectal area. Ultimately, this area will also start sending pain signals, via their nerves, to your brain. It is not uncommon for women to be comfortable for hours with the epidural only to be convinced that it's partially malfunctioning at seven or eight centimeters dilation because they feel increasing pressure again—this time in the vaginal-rectal area.

What's happening? The epidural medication is probably not getting to the vaginal-rectal nerves quite as well as it was getting to the nerves higher up. How well medication spreads downward probably has more to do with your individual anatomy around the epidural space than with the epidural itself.

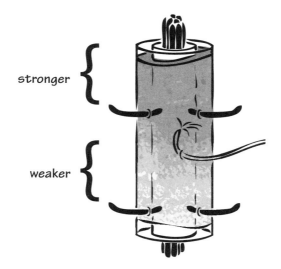

There are complete and partial solutions to the problem. First, a bolus or boluses can be given, pushing some medication down, even if more medication also heads upward. This usually helps immensely. Less often, it at least helps partially.

If your epidural isn't working as well as you or your anesthesiologist would like, occasionally the reason is that, although everyone did their best, your epidural catheter is just too high, or just too much to one side. What to do? Well, if you are willing, the anesthesiologist can replace your epidural and perhaps place it a little lower or a little more to the right. Yes, it's the procedure again, but at this point you will have been through it once before, and you will realize that it isn't much of an ordeal.

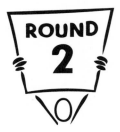

Finally, despite the ridiculous amount of tape we put on your back, and despite all your best efforts, the catheter might fall out, although this is uncommon. To help keep the catheter from dislodging, you will want to avoid in-bed yoga routines or

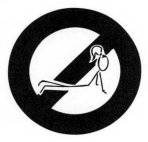

scratching that itch on your back by wriggling against the sheets. To keep the tape in place, be sure you do *not* use moisturizer on

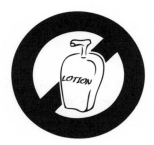

your back before you go to the hospital. The tape won't stick very well to your skin if your skin is moisturized, and if the tape doesn't hold the catheter in place, the catheter may slip out, and you may need to get a second epidural.

I included this chapter, "The Imperfect Epidural," because although most epidurals are administered easily and work well, not all epidurals are perfect. It's good to know why not—and what your anesthesiology team can do about it.

Chapter 7

Side Effects

*A*FTER EXPERIENCING THE BEGINNING part of labor, many women start to consider having an epidural or a spinal but aren't quite committed. They often express how concerned they are about the risks to themselves and to their baby.

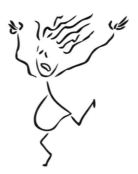

It is amazing how much misinformation there is about such a safe procedure. I can guess where some of it is generated. One source is anesthesiologists and their style of communication. A few anesthesiologists feel compelled to emphasize extremely rare problems, and others leave out expected normal occurrences. The latter have a "less is more" philosophy when it comes to details. But it usually takes only a couple of extra minutes to provide a thorough explanation of the procedure without going overboard. The benefit is that if something should happen, you won't become alarmed but will say to yourself, "Okay, there's nothing drastically wrong. My doctor said this might happen, and it did. No big deal."

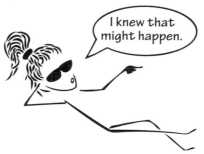

One simple way to think about epidural risks is to relate them to the risks of flying, a common activity where you also put yourself in someone else's hands. Side effects, like turbulence,

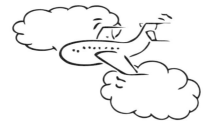

are quite common—even expected—and the anesthesiologist will tell you about them (and I will too, in this chapter). The anesthesiologist will also describe uncommon problems, which are more like finding spilled shampoo in your favorite piece of luggage—it doesn't happen often, but when it does, it temporarily causes you some inconvenience. Problems that occur uncommonly are discussed in chapter 8. Chapter 9 is about rare complications, equivalent to the flying risks you might see in the movies—they happen so rarely that the risk isn't going to stop you from flying down to visit your Aunt Bessie this summer.

All the side effects, common and uncommon problems, and rare complications that I discuss in this chapter and in chapters 8 and 9 also apply to spinals. As I've noted before, think of spinals as almost the same as epidurals. (We will get into the subtle differences for spinals in chapter 11.)

Let's start by briefly talking about the *side effects* of the epidural, those we expect to happen. Even if you're a person who prefers not to know anything about risks, it's a good idea for you to read the next couple of pages. The facts will likely calm your fears rather than stir them up.

Once an epidural is placed and you get the full dose of medication, you can expect to have a *warm, tingly, and even numb sensation in your legs and weak control over your legs.* Recall from

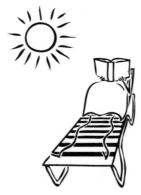

the last chapter that the medication affects not only your pain nerves but also your muscle and temperature nerves. When these latter nerve signals are blocked, your muscles get weak and you feel warm.

Although anesthesiologists care only about sensations (pain signals) from the uterus-cervix and vaginal-rectal areas, we also wind up blocking pain signals from nearby nerves in the epidural space. Those nerves are from your legs and belly. If you feel numb or tingly in any of these places, you shouldn't worry—the epidural is behaving just as it should.

Now, the next side effect. It happens all the time, and
it will happen to you: *your blood pressure will decrease.*
Surprisingly few doctors even mention this side effect,
and then, when it happens, the woman is unnecessar-
ily terrified because if it drops low enough, the health
care team will scurry around the room to fix it.

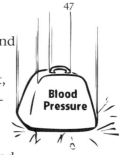

Your team will prepare for the decrease in blood
pressure by first insisting that you get hydrated before
or during the epidural. The liter or more of IV fluid I mention in
chapter 4 does the job of hydrating you—filling you with fluids.
After the epidural is in place, when you lie back down, you will
be purposely tilted to one side or the other. This takes the weight

of your baby and your uterus off one of your main blood vessels,
which circulates your blood back to your heart. It also happens
to take the weight off the major blood vessel feeding your uterus,
so in general, it's a great position to be in.

When your blood pressure drops, it is a good sign that your
epidural is going to work well. The converse is *not* true: if your
blood pressure decreases only a little, you will still likely have a
well-functioning epidural.

In about one out of four epidurals, despite all precautions, the
woman's blood pressure decreases enough to make the anesthesiologist uncomfortable, or to make the woman feel a little dizzy,
or even to make her baby's heart rate slow temporarily. This happens ALL THE TIME. We expect it, and we often stand around
waiting for it to happen, partly to assure ourselves that the epidural is going to work, and partly to counteract, if necessary, the
decrease in blood pressure.

Any or all of the following will happen. A medication to temporarily boost your blood pressure will be given through

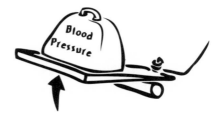

your IV. The medication is a kind of mini-adrenaline and will possibly make your heart race for a short time. Simultaneously, the nurse may ask you to turn in any number of different positions, but usually just to lean all the way to the left or right. He or she might also place some form of extra oxygen on you, give you more IV fluid, and ask someone from the obstetric team to check the dilation of your cervix.

Despite this temporary dip in blood pressure, the pain control from the epidural usually improves the overall blood flow to the uterus and therefore to the baby. This may be why studies could find no deleterious effect of epidurals on newborns when researchers looked at five-minute APGAR scores,[6] umbilical cord blood tests,[7] and neurobehavioral tests of infants.[8] (These specific studies are described in detail in chapter 15.)

Another sometimes worrying reaction is *feeling tired* after *you get complete pain relief.* This is simply exhaustion. Expectant

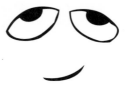

moms often don't realize how exhausted they will be from even the earliest stages of labor. Labor can start any time, like 2 A.M. You start with the excitement, the telephone calls, and the *rush* to the hospital—and then pain keeps you from getting any rest at all, much less sleep. (Even worse, at the hospital they deprive you of your double espresso mocha latte—unforgivable yet true.) Once the epidural's finished, you're exhausted, pain free, and anxiety free . . . and it's time for you to take a well-deserved and much needed nap.

The last side effect you may feel is an *itchy face*. Many people associate itchiness with the first sign of an allergic reaction. That

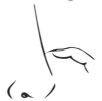

may be true, but if all you experience is itching and nothing else, then it's caused by an additional medication that is usually added to your epidural—a narcotic.

The "-caine" medication, usually bupivacaine or ropivacaine, is the main epidural or spinal medication, and it's responsible for almost all your pain relief as well as most of the side effects, except itchiness, which is from the narcotic. The narcotic is usually called "something-fentanyl" (like fentanyl or sufentanyl), and it's given along with the "-caine" medication because it helps a little with the pain relief—enough so that the strength of the "-caine" medication can be decreased. The less of the "-caine" anesthetic you have, the fewer side effects, like weak legs, you will experience from that anesthetic. For some people, the narcotic makes their whole body itch, not just their face. Most people don't experience this, but a handful of people who are extremely sensitive to the narcotic do. For those few women, we can change the epidural medication to the "-caine" medication only.

Chapter 8

◆

Uncommon Problems

THE BEST WAY TO start a discussion on risk is to first put to rest some common misperceptions about epidurals. Then I'll talk about real issues to consider in making an informed decision.

I've already addressed several misperceptions, but let's recap. In chapter 5, I explained that the epidural catheter is *not* put into

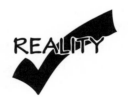

a nerve or into the spinal cord, but is placed into the *compartment* where nerves reside. If a woman moves even moderately during placement, she will *not* be paralyzed. I also pointed out that epidurals *don't* significantly slow down labor, except for possibly creating a little more pushing time at the end.[9] Finally, in chapter 6, I described how and why an epidural may stop working fully, but emphasized that the problem is easily fixable.

Another common misconception is that epidurals can cause back problems after delivery. Many women don't realize that pregnancy itself greatly changes the anatomy of the spine. The natural curvature of the spine becomes exaggerated to offset the frontal weight of the growing baby; the pelvic bones, which

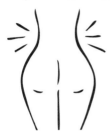

form the base of the spine and the structure of the birth canal, change too. Many ligaments supporting the uterus are attached internally to the lower back—and they, obviously, need to adjust as well.[10] All these changes are necessary to accommodate the passage of the baby, and any of them may contribute to back pain later.

Nonetheless, it's understandable that a woman who has a needle stuck in her back would think that this procedure has something to do with her lower back pain afterward, especially if she doesn't know about how pregnancy affects her back. It's a fair question: Do epidurals have any effect, positive or negative, on after-delivery back problems?

Very large studies were conducted to find out the answer to just that question. These studies looked at literally thousands of women who either received or did not receive an epidural dur-

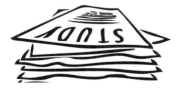

ing childbirth. Researchers found a high incidence of lower back pain after delivery: about one in four women reported having it. The studies did not, however, show any correlation between the back pain and the epidural.[11] In other words, you have the same likelihood of developing lower back pain after pregnancy whether or not you receive an epidural.[12] Of course, any persistent or progressively worsening pain should always be brought to the immediate attention of your obstetrician.

The last big misperception is that epidurals cause a higher rate of Cesarean (C-section) deliveries.

For various reasons, some laboring women who intend to have a vaginal birth need to have a C-section. Two reasons are that the cervix stops dilating or the baby stops descending through the birth canal. Could an epidural placed during labor contribute to this problem? After all, epidurals do somewhat affect a mother's strength. This hypothesis seems logical.

Many years ago, well-meaning doctors tried to figure this out. They compared a large number of women who'd received epidurals to a large number of women who had not received epidurals during their labors. They discovered that women in the epidural group had their delivery plan changed to a C-section more frequently than the women who did not receive an epidural. The investigators concluded that epidurals had some negative effect. Were they right? Not quite. Understanding this misperception involves understanding how medical studies are properly done.

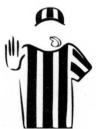

What they neglected to do was "control" the studies. This simply means that the judges didn't make sure all the contestants were equal before starting the race.

When the studies were done, epidurals weren't as popular as they are today. The few mothers in the study who had received epidurals were generally in much more pain *earlier* in their labor. Women experiencing this earlier, significant labor pain tended to have a reason for experiencing such pain. Sometimes the baby was in a bad position for labor and delivery, and sometimes the baby was just too big for the mother's birth canal. Many of the reasons for early or significant pain were also reasons not only for an epidural for pain relief but also for a C-section to deliver a baby who just wasn't going to fit through the birth canal. In

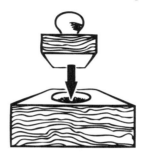

other words, in most of these cases, the underlying reason for the C-section was the same underlying reason that resulted in the woman receiving an epidural.

Since these studies were conducted, multiple higher-quality studies have proved that epidurals have no impact on whether a woman will get a C-section.[13]

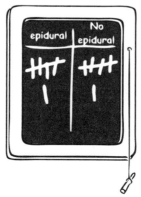

Having said that, everything in life has some benefit and some risk associated with it, and epidurals and spinals are no exception. Fortunately, most women in labor can expect an uneventful epidural or spinal with no adverse effects. The risks to consider are these: the epidural may not work perfectly (discussed in chapter 6); there are some possible side effects (discussed in chapter 7); there's a 1 to 2 percent chance of getting a nasty headache following the epidural or spinal; and epidurals may increase your body temperature. Let's delve into these last two issues right now.

The headaches some women get after epidurals (and after spinals, which I'll discuss in more detail shortly) have a few different names. Technically, they're called "postdural puncture headaches," and unofficially they're called "spinal headaches," even if they result from an epidural.

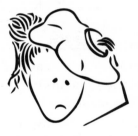

Our goal with the epidural is to place the tip of the epidural needle into the compartment (epidural space) so we can thread the epidural catheter in. If we go a little farther than we intend to go, the needle will poke through the membrane just beyond the epidural space. This membrane holds in the fluid that surrounds the spinal cord. Sometimes we enter this space intentionally when we do a spinal anesthetic (see chapter 11). If we do, what happens?

The problem is with the size of the hole we leave behind. Even though the hole will seal itself, a little fluid still leaks out while it is sealing. The bigger the hole, the bigger the leak. If enough fluid leaks into the epidural space, the woman will develop an unusual headache within a couple of days.

If you receive a spinal anesthetic, which is the anesthetic often used in C-sections and occasionally for labor pain, a hole

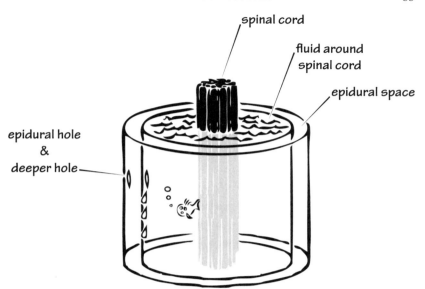

spinal cord

fluid around
spinal cord

epidural space

epidural hole
&
deeper hole

is made in this membrane on purpose. A spinal needle is ultra-thin compared to an epidural needle. This is because a spinal needle only has to allow liquid medication to flow into the fluid around the spinal cord, but an epidural needle has to be large enough to allow the epidural catheter to be threaded into the epidural space. (I discuss the advantages and disadvantages of spinals vs. epidurals in chapter 11.) The hole from the ultrathin spinal needle is tiny, and therefore very, very little fluid leaks out. With spinals there is a one or two in a hundred chance of leaking enough fluid to get this headache.

On the other hand, if you get an epidural and the anesthesiologist places the epidural needle a little farther than intended, he or she might make a similar hole in this membrane, only wider because the epidural needle is wider. In this situation, you will almost definitely get the headache. About one in every one hundred women getting an epidural gets this headache as a result. The incidence of a spinal headache from an epidural and a spinal headache from a spinal are about the same. The bottom line is that if you're getting an epidural or a spinal, there's a 1 to 2 percent chance of experiencing a spinal headache.

Spinal headache symptoms are unique. The headache worsens when you sit or stand up and greatly improves when you lie down. Other symptoms may go along with these headaches, too, like a stiff or sore neck, nausea, and eye irritation in bright light. In rare cases, women develop double vision or hear strange sounds, like ringing or buzzing. A doctor, not you, should determine whether you have a spinal headache, because your symptoms could be related to something more serious.

The symptoms are at their worst a couple of days after the procedure and usually go away on their own over a few days as the hole seals itself. Most people get relief from drinking a moderate amount of fluid, particularly caffeinated beverages. I usually advise women to try drinking plenty of caffeine early in the day, when they need to be upright more, then noncaffeinated fluids later. This way they can actually fall asleep when the symptoms disappear because they're lying flat. New mothers with a spinal headache can also take mild analgesics like ibuprofen or small doses of stronger pain killers to tide them over until the headache goes away, but any medications must first be okayed by their obstetrician.

For most people with spinal headaches, fluids, caffeine, and pain medications suffice until the headache goes away. When

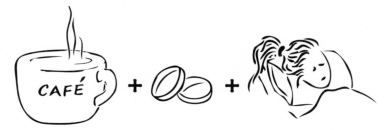

this approach does not help, a more definitive treatment called an "epidural blood patch" will. This procedure can be done as early as twenty-four hours after the hole is created and is usually performed before the woman leaves the hospital. Some women try fluids, caffeine, and medications at home and then change their minds and come back to the hospital for a few hours to have the epidural blood patch.

An epidural blood patch is just like the epidural, as described in chapter 5, with a couple of exceptions. The first is that the anesthesiologist will need to draw blood from your arm. Then, instead of threading in the epidural catheter, he or she will inject your own blood back into your epidural space. This literally patches the hole. Although the blood patch is another procedure to undergo, it has an incredibly high success rate. One study concluded that the blood patch was 75 percent completely effective and 18 percent partially effective. The failure rate was the remaining 7 percent.[14]

The choice of whether to get a patch is generally up to you if you're the one or two in a hundred women who get this headache. Sometimes there is no choice, and the epidural blood patch has to be done, such as if you develop the unusual symptoms of double vision or ringing or buzzing in your ears.

A few serious obstetric problems cause headaches too. Even if you're sure a headache is related to an epidural or a spinal, promptly discuss it with your OB doctor and team.

Laboring women, for numerous reasons, may experience an increase in their body temperature. If that temperature breaks

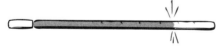

100.4°F (or 38°C), then it's called a "maternal fever." Maternal fevers have been associated with many factors, including long labors, first-time mothers, infections, and, most recently, labor epidurals.

How labor epidurals cause an increase in temperature is still unclear. One possible explanation has to do with both shivering and sweating. Normally the body shivers to produce heat and sweats to rid itself of heat. Laboring women may shiver even when they are not cold. For reasons we don't understand, this shivering occurs most commonly in first-time laboring mothers. Shivering is even more common if the woman has a labor epidural. Epidurals also decrease sweating. Thus, the increased heat produced from shivering may be exaggerated when the epidural decreases the body's ability to rid itself of that extra heat through sweating.[15]

Research has linked labor epidurals to maternal fever only in women delivering for the first time. About one in ten laboring women develops a fever during her first labor. With an epidural, the incidence is about one in four.[16] The rise in body temperature associated with an epidural, if it occurs, is usually small and develops over hours. There is no direct negative consequence of a maternal fever if it is solely due to an epidural. Fevers from epidurals are *gradual*. First-time mothers, on average, have *longer labors* compared with mothers delivering for a second or third time. One theory is that the longer the epidural is in place, the more likely it is that the expectant mother will break the arbitrarily set line where a temperature is defined as a "fever," or the more likely the change in temperature that occurs will be considered statistically significant.

Some women develop infections before or during labor and delivery. A maternal fever may lead the obstetric team to search for an infection, unless they feel certain the fever is due to the epidural. Concerns about an infection could also cause the medical team to prescribe a short course of antibiotics. Similarly, the baby's pediatrician may take a different approach to the baby's care if the mother had a maternal fever. I look more closely at an epidural's implications for the newborn in chapter 15.

Chapter 9

Rare Complications

*I*F YOU BOARD AN airplane and the pilot warmly greets you at the door and assures you that the airplane has been thoroughly checked out, and that he or she is an experienced pilot, but that there's always an extremely small possibility that the plane will crash, you might be shocked at his or her untempered honesty—but you would probably take the flight anyway. People take tiny risks all the time. Epidurals, spinals, and general anesthetics also involve tiny risks.

Some people like to hear about these rare risks, regardless of how likely or unlikely they are, but most people would rather not. Again, wouldn't you rather take that flight without first hearing from the pilot that there's an infinitesimal chance that the plane will crash? That's why when I discuss epidurals (or any anesthetic) with patients, I automatically tell them about the common and uncommon risks, as I've done in the previous two chapters, but I give them the *option* of hearing about very rare risks. If someone wants to hear them, I continue on, and that's what I'm doing in this chapter, too. I'm giving you that option: feel free to skip this chapter if, like many other people, you would rather not hear about the rare risks. It's perfectly okay to decide that you'd rather not know the details, even if, like with the plane crash example, you've already heard about the rare risks in a general way, in conversations or in the media. If you decide to read the rest of this chapter, rest assured that I'll give you some perspective on the risk so that you can put it into context with things that happen in everyday life.

Of all the rare complications of a spinal or an epidural anesthetic, the most common concern for women is nerve injury that causes paralysis, and therefore nerve injury is the primary focus of this chapter. The concern is, I believe, generated from two sources: one is the public's misconception that a needle is placed into a nerve or into the spinal cord, as I discussed in chapter 5. The other relates to complications that occurred when regional anesthesia was being developed. In other words, there

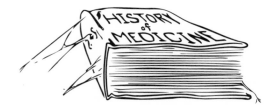

were some problems in the past. For years now, however, those problems have been remedied.

Some women have heard a story related to expensive epidural and spinal needles being sterilized and reused. People receiving epidurals or spinals through those needles were injured because the cleaning agent used to sterilize the needles was apparently toxic to nerves. Residual cleaning agent on the needles caused damage when placed near nerves.

This is no longer a concern at all, because epidural and spinal kits in most of the modern world, including the United States, are one-use sets. This means they are not cleaned—they are thrown away. Everything in the set is *always* thrown out after it's used on a person.

Another problem that occurred in the past is well documented, unlike the cleaning agent problem. When a special "micro" (ultrathin) spinal catheter was introduced, a problem with the distribution of medication occurred and led, infrequently, to permanent nerve damage.[17] These micro-catheters are no longer being used, which means that this problem, too, is no longer a concern.

More recently, but still many years ago, people who had medical problems requiring an extremely powerful blood thinner, such as Coumadin, Lovenox, or Plavix, had bleeding in their epidural space after an epidural or a spinal anesthetic.[18] The bleeding led to permanent nerve damage and, in some cases, paralysis. Now, women who are taking any of these strong blood thinners are not given epidurals or spinals unless they have been off the medication for a specified time.

Although medical procedures have been changed to address problems that happened in the past, there is still an extremely tiny risk of permanent nerve injury from an epidural or a spinal. It is difficult to say exactly how often permanent nerve damage occurs, partly because nerve injury is so infrequent and partly because the studies that find rare problems do not separate nerve injury resulting from an epidural or a spinal from nerve injury resulting from the delivery itself. Injuries during delivery, called "obstetric palsies," occur when the baby, while descending through the birth canal, severely compresses nerves that travel from the lower back to the legs. Unfortunately, these injuries caused by delivery are sometimes confused with injuries caused by anesthesia, and in the end, the epidural or spinal takes the rap.[19]

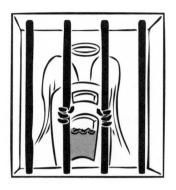

A recent meta-analysis—a study in which many smaller studies are brought together to create one large study—sought to find out how many obstetric patients suffered permanent nerve injury from procedures related to labor and delivery. Researchers looked at a total of twenty-seven studies that met their criteria. This allowed them to consider a total of 1.37 million women who had received epidurals for childbirth. Persistent nerve injury of any degree, even if it was only mild numbness, occurred in approximately 1 in 240,000 patients.[20]

To give you some perspective, consider this risk in the context of the risks you take every day, traveling around. According to a recent year's motor vehicle crash and casualty statistics, there's a 0.0000000113 chance of death for each mile traveled.[21] This means that the likelihood of a person dying in a motor vehicle accident over just a couple of weeks is about the same likelihood of a woman suffering a permanent nerve injury from an epidural for childbirth.[22]

There are a few other rare risks. One is the very small chance that you could develop an infection in the epidural space.

Another is that you could experience an allergic reaction to one or more of the medications we give. These and other rare adverse reactions are nearly always treatable.

As with any medical procedure, the list of truly rare events is long (think about the extensive insert that lists all the possible adverse reactions to your nonprescription medications). If you

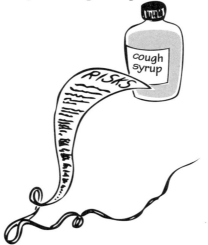

are concerned about something specific, be sure to talk with your medical care team so that they can put your concern in perspective.

Chapter 10

◆

Conditions Affecting
Epidurals and Spinals

$\mathcal{S}$OME EXPECTANT MOTHERS HAVE conditions that
may concern them and their medical team. Some conditions
are unimportant when it comes to epidurals or spinals, but others need to be carefully considered before these procedures are

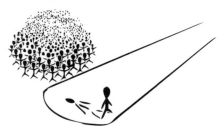

done. A few conditions mean that the woman cannot safely receive regional anesthesia like an epidural or a spinal and should
not have one.

In this chapter I touch on the most common conditions that
cause concern:

> herniated (bulging) discs
> previous back surgery

scoliosis (curvature of the spine)
lower back tattoos
bleeding abnormalities
preeclampsia

Lower back pain is caused by several factors. In chapter 8 I dispel the common misconception that epidurals or spinals cause back pain after childbirth. But what if you had back problems *before* pregnancy? The most common reason we anesthesiologists see a woman in our offices before labor starts is that the woman has a herniated, or bulging, disc (or discs) and is worried about whether she can have a safe and effective epidural or spinal.

Unlike the large studies on labor epidurals and back pain,

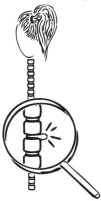

no good studies look only at women with herniated discs who receive epidurals for childbirth. However, doctors have had a great deal of *experience* with epidurals and herniated discs. The epidural procedure is often performed by pain specialists as a treatment for back pain. The main difference between this epidural and the labor epidural is that the medication used to treat back pain is a steroid to decrease the inflammation that is causing pain, instead of a medication to block pain signals related to labor and delivery.

A potential concern arises from the unusual posture a woman gets into during the pushing phase of delivery. The combination of this position and her forceful pushing may aggravate an existing back condition. An epidural will blunt the pain she will feel, so she may not know if she is pushing herself beyond her comfort limit, given her back condition.

What we know is that a vast number of people with bulging discs report no problems from an epidural. When I talk with women who have chronic lower back pain and who have received two or even three epidurals for previous pregnancies, they never indicate that their disc problems got worse from having epidurals. My colleagues tell me that they have also talked with women in this situation, and again, the women report no problems. The collective anecdotal experience of seasoned anesthesiologists, however, cannot replace medical studies, which, to the best of my knowledge, do not exist. How can you make a decision if the medical studies have not been done?

Consider the following. First, we know that the procedure itself should not cause a problem because epidurals are sometimes used to treat chronic lower back pain from bulging discs. Second, if you are getting an epidural or a spinal for a planned C-section (which I discuss in chapter 12), you'll never be in the physical position required for pushing—nor will you be pushing—so physical positioning won't aggravate your back problem. Third, because so many people have bulging discs and have had labor epidurals or spinals, if there were serious problems or if many people had problems, we would expect to see a significant number of reports in the literature—and we haven't.

Nonetheless, without clear guidelines for providing regional anesthesia to laboring women who have herniated discs, different physicians make different decisions about whether to do so. In my experience, most doctors will. I suggest that you contact the anesthesia department through your obstetrician months before your delivery date to assess the severity of your condition. If you meet with the anesthesia team, remember to bring with you any radiology reports (such as x-rays and MRIs) and written reports of your doctor's diagnosis of your condition.

Another common back condition is curvature of the spine, also called scoliosis. Scoliosis will not stop you from having an epidural or a spinal, but it may make it slightly more difficult to place the catheter in an acceptably midline position. (See chapter 6 for a discussion of epidural catheter position problems.)

If you have scoliosis and you are having an epidural, you can assist your anesthesiologist while helping yourself. Even though you won't feel pain during the placement of an epidural (or a spinal), you will feel a little pressure. During the procedure, if you happen to feel pressure a little more to the left or to the right, say so. Even though we aim for what we think is the exact midline of your epidural space, we don't have x-ray vision. I often ask my patients whether they think I'm more to one side or the other, and their answers always help guide me.

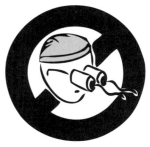

Some women with scoliosis or herniated discs have undergone corrective surgery on their backs before pregnancy. What surgery was done and where on the back the surgery was performed will greatly affect whether you have an epidural space left. If you have had previous back surgery, visit your anesthesiologist well before you go into labor, with previous x-rays and other tests and diagnoses in hand.

Chance favors the prepared mind
Louis Pasteur

It's to your advantage to see the anesthesia team in this situation even if you have no intention of accepting a labor epidural. About one in three planned vaginal deliveries turns out to be a C-section delivery, and the preferred anesthetic for a C-section is a spinal or an epidural rather than a general anesthetic.

On a lighter note, let's chat a bit about body art. Tattoos, particularly lower back tattoos, have become hugely popular. About one in five women of childbearing age has a tattoo. Since tattoos

consist of dye embedded in the skin, there has been concern about passing a needle through this area and possibly introducing the dye into the epidural space.

Some experts believe that fully healed tattoos with fully dry dye are not a problem. They suggest that "dye is inert and even the microscopic amount of skin that might be drawn into the body should pose no risk." But other anesthesiologists remain unsure about accessing the epidural space through tattooed skin. Almost everyone I work with will try to avoid a tattoo and still give the woman her epidural. Two FDA studies are reportedly under way to clarify this issue.[23]

A much more worrisome condition is a bleeding abnormality. There are many causes of bleeding problems. Some stem from

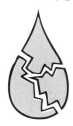

childbirth, and others occur later in life, from some disorder, disease, or medication. In chapter 9 I discussed the potentially disastrous consequences if an epidural or a spinal is placed in a woman with a bleeding abnormality caused by very strong blood thinners. The risk of a serious problem exists with a bleeding abnormality from any cause. This is why a woman with a history of easy bruising or unusually excessive bleeding, or someone who has taken medication or acquired a disease or disorder that may affect her blood's ability to clot, will raise red flags for any anesthesiologist. Very few of the epidurals and spinals out of the

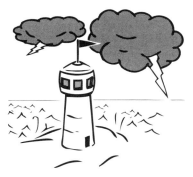

millions administered actually result in nerve injuries, but when a nerve injury does occur, a preexisting bleeding abnormality is often the cause.

Women with a history of easy bruising and women whose blood does not clot easily after an injury need to discuss their history with their obstetricians *early* in their pregnancy. A physician called a hematologist, who specializes in blood abnormalities, can conduct simple blood tests to see if you are at risk of having significant bleeding, which can increase your chances of a nerve injury. Although the tests are simple, it can take days to get the results back. Expectant mothers with this history who

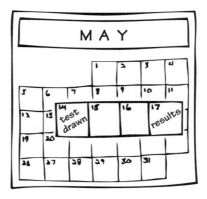

are already in labor and have no blood tests available to reassure their doctors that it's safe to place a regional anesthetic may be refused an epidural or a spinal for labor or may require a general anesthetic if they need a C-section.

The same concern applies to women who are taking strong blood thinners. Weak blood thinners, like aspirin or ibuprofen, *usually* pose no problem, as long as the medication is taken within its guidelines. Some expectant moms develop blood clots in their legs, and these clots are treated with strong blood thinners, typically longer-acting types. These can be replaced by shorter-acting medication (such as heparin) as you near your delivery date. Under the direction of your obstetrician you can stop taking the shorter-acting blood thinners just hours before an anticipated epidural or spinal.

Women taking a holistic approach to their pregnancy will have to be careful about any herbal supplements they use, because some of these supplements can affect the blood's ability to clot.

Last, there is a relatively common pregnancy-related condition called "preeclampsia." This condition, which can affect the blood's ability to clot, typically appears late in a pregnancy and can occur even after the woman goes into labor. Approximately one in twenty women develops this condition.

It is beyond the scope of this book to delve into the details of preeclampsia. If your obstetrician suspects that you have it, you will need a relatively quick blood test before you can receive a regional anesthetic. The test has to be done within a few hours of

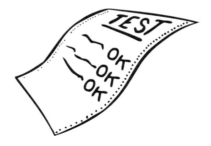

the planned epidural or spinal. The results are often obtainable in about an hour. In our imperfect world, sometimes the timing of "recent enough" blood tests and the inexact timing of your epidural don't coincide. If you're the one in twenty women who develops preeclampsia, raise the need for the blood test with your nurse before or in the first stages of labor and ask to meet the anesthesiologist early.

Chapter 11

Spinals and Walking Epidurals

*A*LTHOUGH AN ANESTHESIOLOGIST won't hand you the equivalent of a fancy martini list to see what you're in the mood for, there are many possible modifications to the typical epidural. You don't need to understand all their subtle

differences, but you may want to know about some of the common variations so you'll be better prepared to encounter them. You can choose to skip most of this chapter, but be sure to read the first part, about spinals, if you know you will be getting a spinal—say, for a planned C-section. On occasion an anesthesiologist will administer a spinal instead of an epidural for labor, so you might want to understand the difference even if you aren't planning on having a spinal for labor and delivery.

Spinals are almost identical to epidurals. The preparation (discussed in chapter 4), the procedure (discussed in chapter 5), and the problems (discussed in chapters 6–10) are roughly the same, with a few exceptions. The spinal needle is much, much thinner than an epidural needle. The epidural needle has to accommodate the epidural catheter, but the spinal needle only has to be big enough to allow the passage of liquid medication for a couple of seconds. The needle size won't matter to you either way, because you'll get the initial numbing medicine *before* any epidural or spinal needle is placed. The spinal needle, however, is purposely placed into and a little beyond the epidural space. It travels through the membrane I describe in chapter 5 and into the fluid surrounding the spinal cord. Please note that it goes into the spinal *fluid*, and *not* into the spinal cord itself. In fact, to avoid a woman's spinal cord, we purposely insert the needle at a level in the back below where the cord is expected to end. For simplicity's sake, I'll refer to this fluid-filled space as the "spinal space."

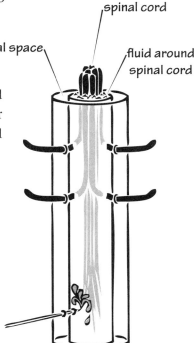

Occasionally, maybe one in ten times, the spinal needle brushes or even bumps into a nearby nerve in the spinal space. If it does, you'll get a temporary shock-like sensation down a leg. The sensation usually goes away in a second or two. Nonetheless, you should tell the person performing the procedure what you are feeling.

For just a spinal, that's really it for the procedure: there's no catheter, no tape. We inject a small amount of medicine into the spinal fluid and then, of course, pull the needle out. The medication floats up and around, distributing itself to all the nearby nerves and to the spinal cord, higher up.

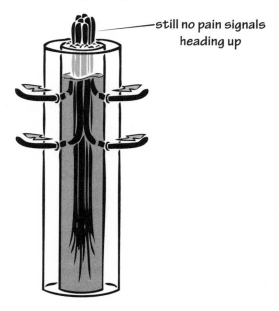

still **no pain signals**
heading up

The spinal medication blocks the nerve signals in a way that is similar to how the epidural medication blocks the nerve signals, but it does behave slightly differently in this compartment. You will almost immediately (meaning within a matter of seconds) feel significant pain relief, including in those harder-to-reach vaginal-rectal areas.

The upsides are that the procedure is quick, and the medication works almost instantaneously. The downsides are that the medication lasts for only a couple of hours and we can't re-dose it—no boluses, no infusions, no little extra dose of pain-numbing medication. Spinals have similar risks as epidurals, including

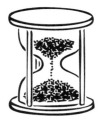

the same 1 to 2 percent incidence of that nasty headache I talked about in chapter 8.

A woman benefits most from a spinal for labor when she arrives for what is at least her third vaginal delivery already dilated to eight or nine centimeters. In this situation we can be fairly certain that she'll deliver within the next hour or two, so the one-shot spinal dose should last long enough to deliver her baby. It will also take effect quickly enough if she delivers within ten minutes.

Although an epidural can't compare with the spinal's speed of onset, it trumps a spinal easily in the category of endurance. Remember, we can give epidural medication through the epidural catheter indefinitely. Since the duration of labor is fairly unpredictable, epidurals are more popular than spinals for mothers and their doctors unless the baby will clearly be delivered in less than two hours.

Some of you might be thinking, *Gee, wouldn't it be nice if you could get the benefits of a spinal and the benefits of an epidural all wrapped up in one?* A combined spinal and epidural (CSE), also called a walking epidural, is just that. The CSE saves the ten

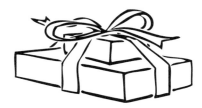

minutes of waiting for a conventional epidural to work, and for a relatively short time, it allows you to walk around a bit . . . hence the name walking epidural. If you do walk, you will need assistance so that you don't trip and fall. The walking epidural may affect the "positioning senses" of your feet in a similar way to the conventional epidural.

The procedure is literally a combination of the epidural and spinal procedures. Just after the epidural needle tip is placed into the epidural space, and just before the epidural catheter is threaded into place, a spinal needle is inserted through the wider epidural needle. The extremely thin spinal needle is slightly longer than the epidural needle and is able to pop out of the epidural needle tip into the epidural space and move a couple of millimeters deeper, into the spinal space.

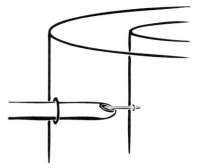

Just like with a spinal, medication is injected into the spinal fluid and works instantly. Then the spinal needle is removed, and the epidural catheter is threaded into the epidural space as if the spinal part never happened. Now you get that super fast pain relief, and when the spinal medication wears off, the epidural catheter is in place so that the anesthesiologist can give a bolus, or add medication, as described in chapter 6.

Some anesthesiologists swear by walking epidurals; others aren't as enthusiastic about them. I won't get into all the nuances of why. Ultimately, you won't get much of a choice because the great benefits and very small risks of each are similar. Instead, expect your anesthesiologist to do what's best for you depending on your individual circumstance.

Some institutions are starting to add devices to the epidural pumps that allow you to self-administer boluses, if and when you need them. This means that you do not have to wait for someone like yours truly to show up with the additional medication. This convenience is called "patient-controlled epidural analgesia," or PCEA. (You know doctors. They have to have an acronym for everything.)

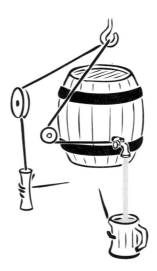

You get the same strength of medicine each time you administer an extra dose to yourself, and the dose is programmed to be a certain amount, with built-in limits. If your self-administered boluses aren't helping enough, you may still need someone like me to administer extra medication. (Hey, sometimes it's nice to be needed.)

Chapter 12

Anesthesia for C-Sections

*A*SURGICAL DELIVERY, or Cesarean section, also known as a C-section, is an extremely common way of giving birth. The number of babies being born this way is steadily increasing. At the time of this publication, the national C-section rate is about one in three deliveries and rising.[24]

Women need to deliver by C-section rather than vaginally for a host of reasons. For example, an expectant mother's obstetrician will know in advance if her ballerina-sized birth canal is not going to accommodate her football player–sized child. Or perhaps a mother-to-be is in the midst of labor and the baby isn't responding well— in that case, the baby has to be delivered in a hurry, without undergoing any additional stress. Maybe the baby is breech, meaning positioned in the uterus sideways or with his or her bottom facing down.

Probably half the women who plan on a vaginal delivery and deliver by C-section instead are unhappy about it. They were mentally prepared for a vaginal delivery, not a C-section. But

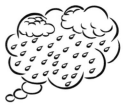

try to keep a couple of things in mind. First, it's *not your fault* if you need a C-section. When someone puts so much effort into one outcome and gets another, feelings of inadequacy sometimes result. As your OB doctor can tell you, the decision for a C-section is almost always made on medical grounds. Second, please appreciate that C-sections have not been around forever. In the old, old days, if the baby couldn't be born vaginally, the baby and the mother would both perish. Fortunately, today we have this very safe and time-proven technique available for both mother and child.

Anesthesia for a C-section is either general anesthesia, which puts you to sleep, or regional anesthesia, given in the form of an epidural or a spinal.

Both general and regional anesthetics are *safe*; however, in most situations, regional anesthesia (a spinal or an epidural) is

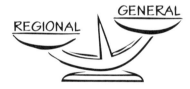

safer for both you and your unborn baby. (In chapter 15 you'll find a more detailed safety comparison between general and regional anesthesia with respect to the baby's well-being.)

Your anesthesiologist will always use his or her best judgment in choosing the appropriate anesthesia for your given situation. Anesthesiologists always lean toward using a regional anesthetic if the situation allows it. Let's discuss this approach first.

Operations happen in an operating room (OR), the safest, most sterile environment in which to have surgery. Labor happens in

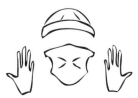

a different kind of environment—in a labor and delivery (L&D) room, which is often warm and homey for the expectant mother and her family and friends. A C-section—which is, after all, an operation—requires a spotlessly clean setting. Granted, an OR isn't as cozy as an L&D room, but your medical team will make some exceptions that they wouldn't make for another kind of operation. The most important one, usually, is that your significant other, a parent, or a friend can be there with you. You might be able to have a little background music, but there's no mood lighting (the medical team needs bright lights). Nearly everyone in the room is usually upbeat, because they like to be around babies being born. (On occasion a tired, grouchy doctor or nurse might sneak in. Just ignore them.)

If the plan for your delivery changes from a vaginal delivery to a C-section and you already have an epidural in place because you had been laboring toward a vaginal delivery, then you are all set. If you do not have an epidural in place, then the anesthesiologist will place a spinal or an epidural once you arrive in the OR.

Spinals and epidurals, as I've emphasized, are practically identical. They are as described in chapters 5 and 11, with only one major difference: the medication we use for a C-section is significantly stronger than the medication used for labor.

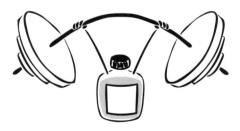

Once your doctor determines that you need a C-section, the staff, including your anesthesiologist, will interview you. The interview will usually happen someplace other than in the operating room you'll be going to shortly. You will sign multiple forms. An IV will be started, and you'll be given that liter of IV fluid described in chapter 4. The preparation differs slightly at this point from the preparation for a labor epidural. Before a C-section, you will receive a couple of medications in your IV and a shot-glass amount of liquid antacid to drink.

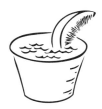

You'll only enjoy the drink if you're especially fond of sucking on limes. The antacid is essential, because the acid in your stomach has to be neutralized to make the anesthesia for the surgery safer. All the fuss has to do with any food or drink in your stomach. A completely empty stomach is ideal, which is why you would be asked not to eat or drink for eight hours before a planned C-section. Whether you have been NPO (*nil per os*, in Latin, meaning "nothing by mouth") or not, the acidity of anything hanging around in your stomach is minimized by this lemony-limey drink and the IV medications.

Some women decide to have their morning coffee anyway, even though they know they are having a planned C-section later that day. Although it's hard to imagine that a little coffee could cause a problem, the fact is that the "starvation rule" is in place solely for your safety. We take it seriously, and we will postpone your *planned* C-section without hesitation, because we're so invested in optimizing your safety. Of course, this rule is broken for an urgent C-section.

When the medical team has all their ducks in a row, the nurse will escort you into the operating room. If you've never been in an OR, it's sure to take you slightly by surprise. Operating rooms all seem a little too chilly and a little too bright, at least initially. Extra staff members are often in the room, and you may be surprised to see so many people. The bed will seem oddly narrow to you. No one expects you to be cool as a cucumber. It's absolutely normal for you to feel apprehensive about all this. Even though everyone in the OR is usually a seasoned veteran, they understand that you're certainly not.

Once you are in the OR and settled, they'll put some monitors on you: a blood pressure cuff, a sticker on a finger, some EKG pads. None of these monitors will hurt you in the slightest.

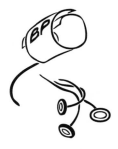

If you don't already have an epidural in place, then at this point the nurse will help you get in position for the epidural or spinal (as discussed in chapter 5): Remember how you need to curl your back like a cooked shrimp?

The epidural or spinal proceeds as described in chapters 5 and 11. The anesthesiologist will clean your lower back with a cold solution and insert the very small needle with numbing medication (which will sting for five seconds). You'll feel a little pressure from the epidural or spinal needle and a possible one-second shock-like sensation down a leg, then the medication being placed in the epidural or spinal space, and the needle being removed. Then they'll quickly lay you down flat to assure the epidural or spinal medication spreads evenly.

Recall that for a vaginal delivery, you don't want the nerve signals from your abdominal muscles and legs to be blocked (as discussed in chapter 6). But if you're getting a C-section, you won't care about your abdominal muscle strength because you won't need to push a baby out through your vagina. Your obstetrician doing the surgery, however, *wants* those nerve signals blocked because it is easier for him or her to perform the C-section. Once the medication fully takes effect (in anywhere from two to ten minutes), it may be difficult or impossible to move your legs until the medication dissipates, hours later.

If you already have an epidural in place from laboring toward vaginal delivery, you'll simply get the extra-strong medicine through the epidural catheter upon entrance to the OR. No repeat procedure is necessary.

As the medication takes effect, the team will tilt you partially onto your side and give you extra oxygen through a mask or a thin tube that rests just under your nose. Your anesthesiologist checks how much of your belly is numb. Your arms are stretched out on a couple of arm boards, because there's really no place else for your arms to go. A nurse will clean your belly with antiseptic, and sterile paper drapes will be placed, which creates a visual barrier between your upper body and your lower body.

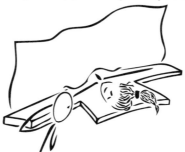

You and your significant other won't be watching the surgery. Most hospitals forbid this, and I seriously advise against it. Some expecting partners really want to watch, though. If your significant other is like this, the staff will point out that there is something even more important—to focus on you and support you while you both experience the birth of your child. Occasionally, partners (or another family member in the OR for support) get overwhelmed or see something that causes them to take a nosedive to the floor. Fainting episodes always seem to occur with men who are most insistent that nothing bothers them. They also tend to be six-foot-two and 220 pounds, which makes them extremely difficult to catch, although I've gotten better at it. I'd prefer to spend all my medical expertise on *you*! Your medical team will try to keep your birth partner sitting with one hand in yours and the other hand on the camera, ready to capture your special moments with the baby, not your body.

You will be awake and feel movement during the C-section. You won't feel any pain from cutting, but you'll feel some pulling and pushing that some women describe as a little uncomfortable. Once they realize that it's normal to feel this movement, most of them are fine with it. Other things you may or may not feel are shivering, a slight heaviness in your chest, and temporary nausea or dizziness. If you don't feel well, please don't be shy. *Tell your anesthesiologist.* Nausea and lightheadedness are common immediately after a regional anesthetic, and they're easily and quickly treatable.

Many women have some doubt that the spinal or epidural can really prevent them from feeling the surgery. It is uncommon for the spinal or epidural to be only partially effective. It is completely normal to have some sensations. For instance, you might feel pressure when the nurse initially washes your stomach area. But please know that the medical team wants you to be numb for the procedure just as much as you want to be numb. For their own reassurance, they do test you (often secretly, without telling you) before they start the surgery, so by the time they start, they're confident that all is well.

Once the obstetrician starts the procedure, most women relax. Some even doze off, especially if they have been in labor for a long time or have been pushing to deliver before the C-section was decided on. Some expectant mothers ask for sedation in addition to the epidural or spinal anesthetic. The IV sedation medications we give are generally inconsequential to the baby, but most physicians prefer to delay giving them until after delivery, because a tiny amount does circulate to the baby if it's given to the expectant mother *before* the baby is born. For those few women with a partially functioning regional anesthetic, extra IV medication will be added to assure their comfort.

A typical C-section takes about forty-five minutes, but durations vary greatly. Getting your baby out is usually the shorter part of the procedure, and fixing you back up perfectly is the longer part. Your obstetrician will answer any questions you have about the specifics of the C-section.

Just before delivery, you'll feel the most pushing on the top of your belly. Once your baby is born, your obstetrician may or may not let you have a quick peek at the baby, depending on his or her own preferences, such as wanting the nurse to dry the baby off right away. Ultimately, you'll see your baby swaddled in a soft blanket in the OR, and usually, your significant other will get to hold the baby next to you.

Once you are nearing the end of the procedure, the staff will kick your significant other out, clean you up, swaddle you too,

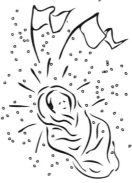

and then transport you via stretcher to the recovery room. This often is the first time you'll be able to hold your baby, possibly breastfeed if you want to, and reunite with family members. Recovery rooms are for recovering from the anesthesia and any after-surgery issues. You won't be allowed to go to your regular hospital room until your regional anesthetic has significantly worn off, any pain or nausea is well controlled, and your obstetric team is happy. Sometimes, it takes hours for the regional anesthetic to dissipate.

Now let's touch on a couple of C-section "niceties" that you might want to talk to the hospital staff about. In a labor and delivery room, you have a lot of control, but you have less control in an OR. Some things, however, might be worth asking for. If you want a certain type of background music and your C-section isn't an emergency, then ask to have your CD played or perhaps have the staff tune in an acceptable radio station. No

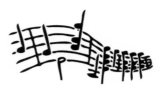

one wants to deliver to Metallica, right? Well, almost no one. It's your delivery and your time. I've never heard doctors or nurses complain or even roll their eyes when someone's made a reasonable request like this.

Another fair request you might choose to make involves your arms. Some anesthesiologists, certainly the minority, feel compelled to secure your arms to the arm boards. These doctors

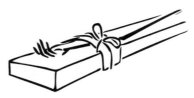

believe they are protecting you from yourself by preventing you from accidentally reaching down under the drapes and into the sterile operative field. Most women, however, prefer to have their arms free. If your anesthesiologist wants your arms secured and you don't, politely say so, but promise to keep your arms where they should be at all times, on your own. You've managed an entire pregnancy; you can certainly handle managing the last two extremities you still have control over for an hour.

General anesthesia is the most common anesthetic for non-obstetric surgery, but it's the least common anesthetic for C-sections. Most anesthesiologists prefer to use regional anesthesia for C-sections, but we're always weighing the benefits and risks of proceeding with one type of anesthetic over another. Sometimes, the best decision for you is to "go to sleep" for your C-section. There are several reasons for deciding that general

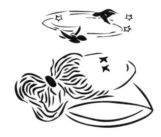

anesthesia is better for a woman. For example, it's difficult or dangerous to place a spinal or an epidural in women with certain bleeding disorders or those with surgical hardware in their back. Occasionally, there's simply not enough time to do a regional anesthetic for an urgent C-section, or the regional anesthetic in place "fails" our test just prior to the start of the surgery.

Preparation for a C-section with a general anesthetic is no different from preparation for a C-section performed with a spinal or an epidural. When you enter the OR, you will lie down, tilt to one side, and have monitors placed on you, as discussed earlier. The oxygen mask will be a little different, and right before you go to sleep, you will feel a couple of fingertips placed gently on your neck.

You'll drift to sleep almost immediately after you receive the medication in your IV. After (and only after) you're asleep, a flexible plastic breathing tube is placed into your mouth and down your trachea (your windpipe). If this sounds unappealing to you, you're not alone in thinking so, but there's no way around it: the breathing tube is inserted for your safety, and you would have one for almost any surgery requiring general anesthesia. At the end of the surgery, as you wake up, the staff will remove this tube. Most people have no memory of having the breathing tube at all. For many women, their first memory after a general anesthetic is of the recovery room.

There is a common misperception that people undergoing general anesthesia initially receive different amounts or types of medication depending on how long the surgery is expected to last. People who have this misperception are understandably concerned that the surgery will outlast the medication, and that they will wake up in the middle of it. What really happens is that throughout the surgery, you receive inhaled medication

continuously, via the breathing tube, so you stay asleep from the surgery's start to finish. The medication is turned off once the surgery concludes, whether that's five minutes or five hours after the surgery began.

Another common concern is the effect of the anesthetic medications on the soon-to-be-born baby. A small amount of any medication, especially IV medication, will get to your baby. But a few facts might lessen your concern. First, the dose of the medication that the baby receives is much smaller than what you get. This is because you break down some of the medication, only a fraction of the medication can cross the placenta to the baby, and the baby starts to break down some of it even before it hits his or her entire circulation.

I rarely observe a "sleepy" baby born via C-section from a mother who has received a non-urgent general anesthetic. Instead, the babies tend to come out kicking and screaming. Also, the type of medications anesthesiologists give you are often the same we'd give the rare newborn who requires surgery within his or her first few days of life. That being said, when regional anesthesia can be done for a C-section, it's still preferable. I address this issue further in chapter 15.

After receiving general anesthesia, you might have a scratchy throat from the breathing tube or nausea from the medication. Before you wake up, you'll likely receive a generous dose of both analgesics (pain medication) and anti-nausea medications that help prevent or minimize pain and nausea during recovery. Occasionally, however, the medications need a little tweaking in the recovery area. Your medical team will make sure you're reasonably awake and comfortable before allowing you to go to your hospital room.

Anesthesia is safer than it has ever been. Whichever type of anesthetic you receive—whether you continue the epidural from an attempted labor, get a spinal in the OR, or receive a general anesthetic—rest assured that your anesthesiologist is trained to make the best choice for you and your baby.

Chapter 13

After Your Delivery

Your EXPERIENCE WITH ANESTHESIA will be over shortly after delivery. Your anesthesiologist will have only a couple of things to do to wrap up. This is good, because by now you'll likely have had just about enough of absolutely everyone except for your baby and perhaps your significant other.

For many new parents, the biggest concern after delivery is figuring out how the nurses perfectly swaddle all the newborns. (I've only mastered how to successfully turn my children into little blanket meatballs.) There are a handful of other issues to consider after the birth, however. Part of your recovery involves recovering from the effects of anesthesia. For a vaginal delivery with an epidural or a spinal, recovery simply consists of waiting for the medication to wear off. This typically takes a couple of hours. During that time, someone from the anesthesia team will remove your epidural catheter. This is normally a painless endeavor except for removing the tape from your back. Any other discomfort you feel after a vaginal delivery will usually be addressed by your obstetrician.

A few women are extremely sensitive to the epidural or spinal medication, and for them, it may take several hours for the medication to dissipate. This isn't a problem as long as your sensation and strength continually improve, but it will be less convenient for you.

Anesthetic recovery from a C-section is a little more complicated, because a C-section is surgery. Most likely the C-section will have been conducted with a regional anesthetic that slowly wears off in the recovery room over two to three hours. You likely received an extra drug in your epidural or spinal cocktail when it was first administered, to help you with after-operation pain for twenty-four hours.

This added spinal or epidural medication is a tiny dose of a long-acting narcotic. Narcotics in the spinal or epidural space don't numb you like the "-caine" medications, and therefore they shouldn't hinder the return of feeling to your belly and legs.

You need to know a couple of things about a C-section recovery. First, the spinal or epidural narcotic you receive might make you a bit itchy or nauseated. Second, although the narcotic will greatly help control the pain, it probably won't get rid of absolutely all the pain you experience. In most hospitals doctors place preset orders in your chart for medications that will help with itching, nausea, and pain, so you'll need to describe what you're feeling when you need help with any of these problems.

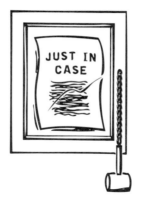

In other words, if you feel itchy, nauseated, or achy, say so. It's not complaining; it's communicating.

More than one type of medication is available to treat each of these problems—itching, nausea, and pain. If one medication doesn't make you feel better in, say, thirty minutes, then request another type. For example, there are at least three different anti-nausea meds. If one type doesn't work, you should get a second one. A second and different anti-nausea medication will work even better than doubling up on the original.

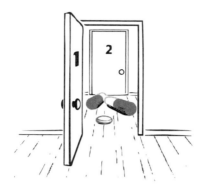

Occasionally, despite all efforts, you just can't get comfortable. Everyone is different, but uncontrollable itching, nausea, or pain is never acceptable. If the medicines you're given aren't

helping, ask your nurse to have your obstetric or anesthesia doctors address your problem promptly.

Approximately twenty-four hours after a
C-section, that tiny dose of spinal or epidural long-
acting narcotic will wear off. If you are experiencing
any side effects, they will go away once this
narcotic is out of your system. However, your
need for supplemental pain medications may
increase slightly at this point.

If you've had general anesthesia for a C-section, you can expect to receive pain medication too, but through your IV. Some
women are given a device that allows them to self-administer
the drug, within set limits. This is called patient-controlled analgesia (PCA).

Regardless of how they are delivered, the pain medications
you receive at this point are narcotics, which means you could
experience itching, nausea, or not quite enough pain relief.
Contingency medications are available to treat all of these. Feel
free to ask for them.

Every once in a while, a woman expresses concern about receiving "narcotics" or "morphine" because she is worried about
becoming addicted to a substance. After any surgery, pain treat-

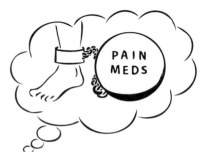

ment comes in some combination of four types of medications.
One is the residual effects of a regional anesthetic, as we've
discussed. Then there's Tylenol, great mostly for headaches.

Nonsteroidal anti-inflammatory drugs (NSAIDs), such as Advil or Motrin, are a helpful addition but don't usually do the trick alone. Finally, there are narcotics, like morphine and oxycodone. It is difficult for most people to get by after surgery by taking only Tylenol or NSAIDs. For the average person, narcotics, used appropriately in this setting, should pose no risk of addiction.

There are uncommon and rare side effects and risks involved with taking any medication, but these issues are beyond the scope of this book. Talk to your doctor if you have any specific questions about pain or pain relief after your delivery.

Chapter 14

Alternatives to Epidurals

*T*HERE MUST BE AT least a dozen different ways to deal with labor pain other than receiving an epidural, and many are touted as being just as good as an epidural. Not everyone has to get an epidural. Not everyone wants an epidural. Some expectant mothers arrive at the hospital with their cervixes already dilated six or seven centimeters, feeling barely any discomfort. One hour and three pushes later, they are cradling their newborn babies. No needles, medications, special breathing, or yoga maneuvers.

Remember that everyone's labor is different. Babies come in different shapes and sizes, and they're in a different position within wombs that are all distinctively shaped. All these babies will emerge out of uniquely formed birth canals. Different people have different wiring in their internal neurological systems, so they feel things differently. What might be painful for one person may not be painful for another. In short, every woman will have a different birthing experience.

You certainly do not have to accept an epidural. There are reasonable alternatives to an epidural, and these alternatives can often be combined with each other. They can even be used while you are considering whether to get an epidural or a spinal, or while you are waiting for one to be administered. You might find that these pain relief methods are just right for you. This chapter summarizes the alternatives to an epidural, but keep in mind these two caveats: one, some approaches, like Lamaze, require research and preparation months before labor begins. Two, these alternatives may not be available at your hospital.

One alternative to receiving an epidural or a spinal is receiving pain medications injected directly in your intravenous (IV) catheter. Many women question why they automatically get an IV when they are admitted to labor and delivery. When an IV medication is administered, the medication will work quickly because it enters your bloodstream directly. Think for a moment about the everyday medications you take at home. If you take a pill, it's broken down in your stomach and intestine, then absorbed into your blood. It then travels and goes to work to address the problem that prompted you to take the pill in the first place. IV medications work quickly because they skip the whole first part of the process. They don't need to be broken down in the stomach and then absorbed into the blood to work. That means no waiting.

Women benefit from having an IV because the IV allows the medical team to immediately handle situations during labor or delivery that require *quick* treatment. One situation is uncontrolled pain.

IV pain medications are usually narcotics with a long record of relative safety, like morphine, Demerol, fentanyl, Nubain, or Stadol. Narcotics permit a direct form of quick pain relief without the epidural or spinal procedure. Don't be concerned about which narcotic medication you receive, because you probably won't be given a choice of which IV medication you get. Your obstetrician will give you whichever he or she is familiar and comfortable with.

A small amount of all medications you receive while you're laboring, including the IV medication, circulates to your not-yet-born baby. The baby's exposure to medications is usually inconsequential, even for epidurals that go on for hours.[25] Doctors won't limit how much epidural medication you can get (except possibly during the pushing phase, as mentioned in chapter 6), but they will limit your IV medication, especially as you near the birth. The IV medication is limited to minimize the small possibility of making the baby a little sleepy when he or she is born. If this does happen (as it does, though rarely), the baby can be awakened in a number of ways, including by giving him or her an antidote to the pain medication.

IV medications are particularly effective for early labor pain. They will likely make you a little groggy and may cause nausea. They last for a couple of hours and sometimes can be re-administered. Some hospitals offer a PCA device, which connects to your IV and lets you self-administer very small doses of pain meds.

Another alternative to an epidural or a spinal is laughing gas, which is nitrous oxide combined with oxygen. Laughing

gas is breathed in and, like a PCA, is controlled by the patient. Laughing gas is more common in Europe than it is in the United States, and it has a couple of advantages over IV medications. IV

meds are fast, but laughing gas is faster still. It works within seconds, and it provides mild pain relief and euphoria. Its greatest
attribute is that it wears off as quickly as it works, allowing the
woman to control not only how she feels but how long she feels
that way. The gas mixture is reportedly effective in combination
with other alternative methods, like meditation, TENS, or even
IV medications. Yes, it's the same stuff the dentist gives you for
filling that cavity in your sweet tooth.

Transcutaneous electrical nerve stimulation (TENS) is yet another alternative. It involves a harmless device that's connected
to your skin via sticky pads and wires. The device delivers tiny
shocks to your skin wherever the pads are placed. The tingling
sensation that results isn't painful and can interact with your
nervous system to decrease labor pain.

If something like TENS doesn't sound quite aggressive enough
for you, perhaps acupuncture does. Theoretically it encour-
ages your body to release its own endorphins, which function as
naturally produced narcotics. Acupuncture has been shown to
significantly decrease requirements for other forms of pain relief
during labor.[26]

Less invasive modalities include acupressure, massage therapy, and reflexology, none of which involves needles. I can't
imagine massage not being helpful in *any* situation, although
the verdict is still out regarding its proven effectiveness for labor
pain. The same goes for reflexology, which essentially is massage
therapy for the feet. Other pain relief ideas, possibly helpful and
likely harmless, range from aromatherapy (scent) to audio-anal-
gesia (sound).

Some women choose mind-over-body techniques such as
breathing and relaxation exercises, yoga, or hypnosis. Lamaze is
the most popular mind-over-body technique. Laboring women
learn how to relax and how to breathe *with* contractions, which

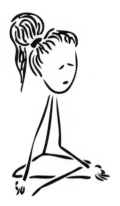

decreases perceived pain. In my experience, Lamaze seems to greatly help most laboring mothers, whether or not they are getting an epidural. Lamaze classes also provide education for parents about pregnancy, labor, birth, and even care for the newborn baby.

Chapter 15

Effects on the Baby

*E*XPECTANT MOTHERS' MOST consistent concern is about what impact medical care will have on their babies.

This chapter focuses on regional anesthesia's potential effects on the newborn. "Regional anesthesia" refers to both epidurals and spinals, and the terms are used interchangeably. Information that is scattered throughout other chapters of this book is compiled here and expanded on.

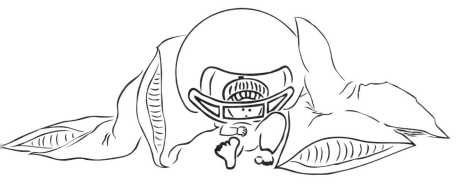

The bottom line is that regional anesthesia has both negative and positive effects on the newborn. The available tests used to assess newborns indicate either no effect to the baby or a possible net benefit to the baby of regional anesthesia in the expectant mother. But let's first delve into the negative aspects.

In chapter 6, I noted that, although epidurals don't slow down dilation of the cervix, or increase the rate of C-sections, they may prolong the pushing phase of delivery by an average of twenty minutes. This may also increase the chance that the obstetrician will want to assist the delivery, such as with the use of forceps.[27] Different obstetricians have different practices when it comes to using forceps. Some will never perform a forceps-assisted delivery; others will use forceps only when the mother has a well-functioning epidural. Studies demonstrate an increased use of forceps in moms with epidurals, but it is unclear whether the epidurals made the forceps necessary or the epidurals gave obstetricians the opportunity to use forceps. Nonetheless, this is one factor to consider.

Epidurals also can increase maternal temperature. The effects of a maternal fever on the laboring mother were addressed in chapter 8. Recall that although there is an increased chance of

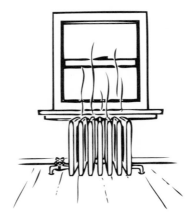

developing a *fever* from an epidural, there is no increased chance of developing an *infection*. Although this bump in body temperature has no known direct consequence, it does tend to confuse the clinical picture for the pediatrician who will ultimately be caring for the baby. The pediatrician may not know whether the increase in temperature was from the epidural, and therefore of no concern, or from some underlying maternal infection that could be transferred to the baby. If there is a significant rise in maternal temperature, the ultimate medical course for the baby ranges from closer observation immediately following delivery to blood tests and antibiotics later. Oddly, fevers are more common with epidurals in first-time mothers.[28]

Epidurals have a few potential advantages to the newborn. Compared with pain medication administered through an IV (as discussed in chapter 14), an epidural or a spinal exposes the baby to much less medication. This is because anything that's injected into the bloodstream of the mother will be shared, to some extent, with the baby. Although IV pain medication's effects on the baby are usually inconsequential, this medication can be eliminated altogether by a labor epidural or spinal. Epidural and spinal pain medication is placed only in the compartment where specific nerves reside (see chapters 5 and 11),

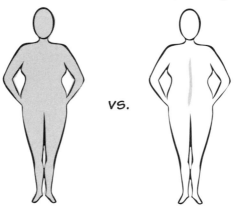

although ultimately even this medication, to some extent, will wind up in the mother's bloodstream. One study examining the effects of labor epidurals on newborns, focusing on fetal drug

accumulation and using special tests on the baby, found no significant adverse effects on the newborn.[29]

Another potential benefit of an epidural relates to the body's
normal reaction to pain. Pain causes the release of the body's
stored natural stress hormones into the bloodstream. These
stress hormones, when released into the maternal blood, will
increase the expectant mother's heart rate and divert blood flow
from her nonvital organs toward her vital organs. Unfortunately,
the uterus, a nonvital organ, doesn't rank very high in this
situation.[30]

In addition, a person in pain tends to involuntarily breathe
quickly; this rapid breathing is called hyperventilation. Hyperventilating decreases the blood's acidity. When a laboring
woman is hyperventilating and there is a resulting fall in the
blood's acidity, the uterus reacts by increasing the resistance to
incoming blood flow.[31]

Because of these two mechanisms—release of stress hormones
and hyperventilation—uncontrolled pain can divert blood
away from the uterus and the placenta, the part of the uterus
where the baby gets his or her oxygen and nutrients. Indirectly
this decrease in blood flow to the mother's uterus will result in a
decrease in blood flow to the baby. Of course, the reverse is also

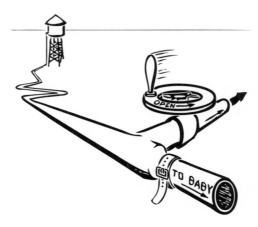

true: treated pain can eliminate this adverse effect. One study measured an increase in placental blood flow after epidurals were placed in laboring women.[32]

Another benefit of a labor epidural involves the anesthetic choices for C-sections. In chapter 12, I noted the increased incidence of C-sections. Many are unplanned, and a portion of them are urgent situations or emergencies.

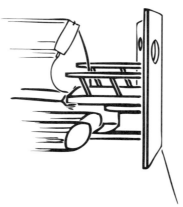

In the world of obstetrics, time is often of the essence. In the world of obstetric anesthesia, a regional anesthetic, meaning a spinal or an epidural, is usually safer for your baby than a general anesthetic.[33] If you're laboring away without an epidural, and suddenly you need a C-section, you will likely have only one choice for an anesthetic: general anesthesia. Why? Because we can do general anesthesia in a fraction of the time it takes to do a spinal or an epidural. But if you have a functioning labor epidural in place, and you suddenly need a C-section, the anesthesiologist can easily use the epidural catheter to give you appropriate pain medication for the surgery. The stronger medication is loaded through the existing epidural catheter. You can be ready for a C-section in usually the same amount of time it would have taken if you'd been given the less desirable general anesthetic.

Now that you know the potentially positive and negative effects of regional anesthesia, you may be wondering about the overall impact on the baby. Several studies have looked into this question. These studies tried to catch differences, positive or negative, in measurable variables between babies born to mothers with epidurals and those born to mothers without. Studies also examine the difference between regional and general anesthesia for C-sections, with respect to the effect on the newborn baby.

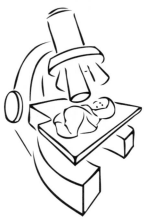

"Measurable variables" are simply things that the medical community believes have some predictive indication of the baby's well-being. They include APGAR scores, neurobehavioral tests, and the acid-base status of the baby's blood.

An APGAR score is a grade the newborn receives at one minute immediately after birth and then again at five minutes after birth. It's based on the infant's heart rate, respiratory (breathing) effort, skin color, muscle tone, and reflex irritability (cry). The high score is ten. Researchers examining APGAR scores found no difference between babies born to women who had received a labor epidural and babies born to women who had not.[34] The usefulness of APGAR scores, however, has been controversial.[35]

In response to this controversy, neurobehavioral testing was developed to, first, provide a more extensive evaluation of the newborn and, second, tease out more subtle differences.[36] There are a few different types of neurobehavioral assessments. All involve a series of tests created to measure a newborn's neurological function and his or her responsive behavior to various stimuli.

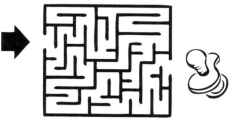

Using the new tests, researchers found no significant difference between babies born to mothers with labor epidurals and babies born to mothers who did not receive any medications for labor.[37] These tests were also used in newborns delivered by C-section. A baby delivered by C-section whose mother had a spinal or an epidural scored significantly better two hours after birth than a baby whose mother required a general anesthetic. This difference disappeared by twenty-four hours.[38]

The last measure is the newborn's acid-base status, which gives us a good idea of what the environment in the uterus was like during labor. If the environment is bad, for numerous reasons beyond this book's scope, the acidity of the baby's blood will rise. The blood's acidity will stay elevated for a short time after delivery and is easily measured. The baby's acid-base status is arguably the best gauge for judging the overall impact of variables during labor—variables like the administration of a labor epidural. In England, one research group combed the literature for studies looking at the effect of labor epidurals versus IV pain medication on the newborn's acid-base status. Their conclusion, after focusing only on what they considered to be quality studies, was that there is a small but significant improvement in acid-base status in babies delivered from mothers who received an epidural.[39] Chapter 16 sums up this discussion—in a nutshell.

Chapter 16

◆

In a Nutshell

*W*HENEVER I MAKE AN important decision about something relatively complex, I try to carefully weigh all the potential advantages and disadvantages. Like most people, I'm a little more mindful when considering something new. Everyone, of course, is different when it comes to tolerance for new things and for risks. I am quite comfortable scuba diving down to sixty feet but quite uncomfortable sky diving from six hundred.

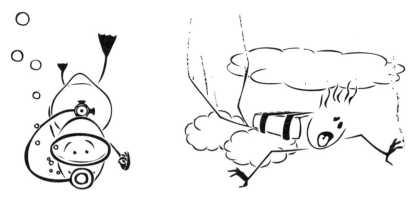

I wrote this book to provide information to help you make a decision and to be comfortable with your decision. How you deal with the pain of labor and delivery is largely in your hands.

I can't be you, and therefore I can't know how you will weigh the relative benefits and risks of accepting regional anesthesia. I do sincerely believe that the advantages are many and great.

And now it's time for admittedly the most biased illustration in this book. Each element of the illustration has been described in previous chapters (and the relevant chapters are noted). I strongly encourage you to read again the section on any of

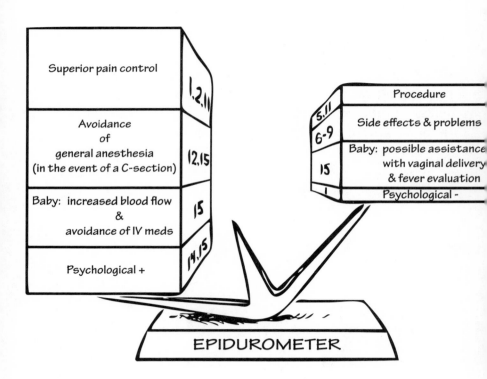

ADVANTAGES   DISADVANTAGES

Superior pain control   1,2,11

Avoidance
of
general anesthesia   12,15
(in the event of a C-section)

Baby: increased blood flow
&   15
avoidance of IV meds

Psychological +   14,15

Procedure   5,11

Side effects & problems   6-9

Baby: possible assistance
with vaginal delivery   15
& fever evaluation

Psychological -   1

EPIDUROMETER

these topics if you need a refresher or if you still haven't made a decision you're comfortable with. Jump back, read, reread, digest, and arrive at your own conclusion.

I hope this book provides you with a painless yet thorough

understanding of the best form of pain relief available to you for labor, as well as a thorough understanding of anesthesia for a C-section. I also hope it helps you understand what is happening to you during your labor, some of the common twists and turns you might encounter, and, more generally, how the process of receiving anesthesia works. May you have a happy and healthy delivery and, most important, a happy and healthy child.

Acknowledgments

$\mathscr{I}$ AM TRULY INDEBTED TO the individuals who contributed their thoughts, perspectives, and time to this endeavor.

I had the incredible good fortune of luring Liliana Naydan, a gifted writer and editor, into the task of balancing this author's nonconformity with the rules of the English language and the laws of common sense. Not only was Lila magnificently successful, but she also skillfully brought clarity to the work while preserving its lighthearted nature. I am convinced the manuscript would never have left my laptop's archives if it were not for her creative and thoughtful contributions.

I am equally indebted to my "unofficial" editors. The very first to set her critical eyes on the work was my everlastingly patient wife, who has painfully put up with me for all these years. Cindy greatly values pursuing life's natural paths while keeping a realistic grip on its boundaries. This, combined with her firsthand experience with the "rough and tumble" of three very different labors, provided me with insight well beyond my reach. She often tried to slow me down "to smell the roses" along my path in writing and publishing this book. I am truly grateful for her desire to do just that, for her encouragement, and for her support. Thank you.

I am truly humbled and honored that both Jacqueline Wehmueller, executive editor of consumer health at the Johns Hopkins University Press, and the Johns Hopkins University Press saw the value in this work and have embraced it as I have. I could ask for no higher honor than that. Jackie has been absolutely wonderful to work with throughout the editorial revisions. Somehow she perfectly balanced candid concerns with gentle guidance, all seasoned with the occasional encouraging praise. Melanie Mallon, the copyeditor, even further enhanced the manuscript. Her patience with all the revisions was greatly appreciated. Sara Cleary, the editorial assistant at JHU Press, was a huge help in guiding me to and through the graphics software. "The enemy of good is better"—I was never sure how exactly to take that expression until I encountered these talented individuals.

The very fortunate and unbelievable chain of events that led to a firsthand introduction to Ms. Wehmueller at JHU Press was facilitated by Martha Murphy. Martha, a writer, an editor, and a book coach, was an invited guest to a Harvard Medical School conference on writing and publishing. It was there that my good luck resulted in the manuscript for *The Epidural Book* stumbling into her hands. Since then, Martha has altruistically guided me. I am forever indebted for that most important connection and for her kind support.

My literary agent, Jeanne Fredericks, was also one of the select few invited guests to the aforementioned Harvard conference. I was impressed with her vast experience, her sincere empathy for the demands placed on medical professionals, and her forthrightness. Jeanne was a natural fit to my personality and a stone's throw away from my home. I am glad she has represented me so well, eloquently being the go-between for many topics and concerns. Jeanne's encouraging words and expert advice have been invaluable.

I owe my sincerest gratitude to my long-time colleagues Drs. Brett Danzer and Raymond Pesso. I am honored they so readily offered their constructive views and were so selfless with their time. I consider myself fortunate to have served side by side with these two remarkable physicians in some of the most trying of circumstances. I cherish their camaraderie and friendship.

Dr. Frederick Lukash, a fellow physician-author, thoughtfully shared his experiences in writing, publishing, and marketing his book, *The Safe and Sane Guide to Teenage Plastic Surgery*. His advice through the publishing world's labyrinth was very helpful.

Professor George Marcoulides, a long-time friend and a rare individual with degrees in both statistics and psychology, was kind to share his expertise in linking risks with everyday life. Stacey Hancock, Ph.D., a statistics professor at my alma mater, Clark University, selflessly combed over my final revisions and verified the conceptual leap from the likelihood of nerve injury from an epidural to the likelihood of fatality while driving. I hope they both use me as a real-life example in their classes of how their discipline reaches nearly every profession.

I'd like to extend my appreciation to North American Partners in Anesthesia (NAPA). I have been quite lucky to find myself ensconced with this assiduous organization by sheer happenstance. NAPA, a rapidly expanding group in the United States, prides itself on high-quality anesthesia services. One component of "high quality" is their continuous quest to expand knowledge beyond the border of the hospital's doorsteps. NAPA's support of this endeavor is one example of their commitment to this cause. I am proud to be a part of this establishment.

I'd be remiss if I didn't briefly touch on my past. My father, through example and encouragement, instilled in me my work ethic. My mother is solely responsible for nurturing a strong admiration for both the field of medicine and the value in relieving suffering. Their unwavering support throughout my education, and these ideals, significantly shaped the physician I am today.

Lastly, I'd like to thank my three children, Brandon, Courtney, and Cole, for sharing their adoring father with some nebulous idea that took an all-consuming shape.

Notes

1. David H. Chestnut, *Obstetric Anesthesia: Principles and Practice*, 3rd ed. (Philadelphia: Mosby, 2004), p. 9.
2. Ibid., pp. 289–90.
3. J. Kupersmith, "Quality of Care in Teaching Hospitals: A Literature Review," *Academic Medicine* 80, no. 5 (2005): 458–66.
4. Gonen Ohel et al., "Early versus Late Initiation of Epidural Analgesia in Labor: Does It Increase the Risk of Cesarean Section? A Randomized Trial," *American Journal of Obstetrics and Gynecology* 194, no. 3 (2006): 600–605.
5. M. Anim-Somuah, R. M. D. Smyth, and C. J. Howell, "Epidural versus Non-epidural or No Analgesia in Labour," *Cochrane Database of Systematic Reviews (Online)* 8 (2010).
6. Ibid.
7. Felicity Reynolds, Shiv K. Sharma, and Paul T. Seed, "Analgesia in Labour and Fetal Acid-Base Balance: A Meta-analysis Comparing Epidural with Systemic Opioid Analgesia," *BJOG: An International Journal of Obstetrics and Gynaecology* 109, no. 12 (2002): 1344–53.
8. Angela M. Bader et al., "Maternal and Neonatal Fentanyl and Bupivacaine Concentrations after Epidural Infusion during Labor," *Anesthesia and Analgesia* 81, no. 4 (1995): 829–32.
9. Ohel et al., "Early versus Late Initiation."
10. Chestnut, *Obstetric Anesthesia*, pp. 25–26.

11. Terrance W. Breen et al., "Factors Associated with Back Pain after Childbirth," *Anesthesiology* 81, no. 1 (1994): 29–34. Charlotte J. Howell et al., "Randomised Study of Long Term Outcome after Epidural versus Non-epidural Analgesia during Labour," *British Medical Journal* 325, no. 7360 (2002): 357–59.

12. Ibid.

13. Chestnut, *Obstetric Anesthesia*, pp. 378–82. Ohel et al. "Early versus Late Initiation."

14. V. Safa-Tisserant et al., "Effectiveness of Epidural Blood Patch in the Management of Post-dural Puncture Headache," *Anesthesiology* 95, no. 2 (2001): 334–39.

15. Christopher M. Viscomi and Theodore Manullang, "Maternal Fever, Neonatal Sepsis Evaluation, and Epidural Labor Analgesia," *Regional Anesthesia and Pain Medicine* 25, no. 5 (2000): 549–53.

16. Ibid.

17. B. K. Ross, B. Coda, and C. H. Heath, "Local Anesthetic Distribution in a Spinal Model: A Possible Mechanism of Neurologic Injury after Continuous Spinal Anesthesia," *Regional Anesthesia* 17, no. 2 (1992): 69–77.

18. James M. Hynson, Jeffrey A. Katz, and H. Ulrich Bueff, "Epidural Hematoma Associated with Enoxaparin," *Anesthesia and Analgesia* 82, no. 5 (1996): 1072–75.

19. Cynthia A. Wong, "Neurologic Deficits and Labor Analgesia," *Regional Anesthesia and Pain Medicine* 29, no. 4 (2004): 341–51.

20. Wilhelm Ruppen et al., "Incidence of Epidural Hematoma, Infection, and Neurologic Injury in Obstetric Patients with Epidural Analgesia/Anesthesia," *Anesthesiology* 105, no. 2 (2006): 394–99.

21. "Fatality Analysis Reporting System Encyclopedia," National Highway Traffic Safety Administration, 2009, www-fars.nhtsa .dot.gov/Main/index.aspx [accessed Oct. 3, 2011].

22. Ibid. Assumptions: Federal Highway Administration 2011 average annual mileage for U.S. drivers aged 20–54 is 15,000 miles/year. Fatality Analysis Reporting System 2009 stats used for all motorists.

23. Information about tattoos is derived in part from Rachel Zimmerman, "Why Some Expectant Moms Are Worried about Tattoos," *Wall Street Journal (Eastern Edition)*, Sept. 18, 2007, D1.

24. Fay Menacker and Brady E. Hamilton, "NCHS Data Brief: Recent Trends in Cesarean Delivery in the United States," *Centers for Disease Control and Prevention*, number 35, 2010, www.cdc.gov/nchs/data/databriefs/db35.pdf [accessed Oct. 3, 2011].

25. Bader, "Maternal and Neonatal Fentanyl."

26. Allison J. Macarthur, "Gerard W. Ostheimer, 'What's New in Obstetric Anesthesia,' Lecture," *Anesthesiology* 108, no. 5 (2008): 777–85.

27. Anim-Somuah et al., "Epidural versus Non-epidural."

28. Viscomi and Manullang, "Maternal Fever."

29. Bader, "Maternal and Neonatal Fentanyl."

30. Chestnut, *Obstetric Anesthesia*, p. 297.

31. Ibid., p. 263.

32. A. I. Hollmén et al. "Effect of Extradural Analgesia Using Bupivacaine and 2-Chloroprocaine on Intervillous Blood Flow during Normal Labour," *British Journal of Anaesthesia* 54, no. 8 (1982): 837–42.

33. T. K. Abboud et al., "Comparison of the Effects of General and Regional Anesthesia for Cesarean Section on Neonatal Neurologic and Adaptive Capacity Scores," *Anesthesia and Analgesia* 64, no. 10 (1985): 996–1000.

34. Anim-Somuah et al., "Epidural versus Non-epidural."

35. Chestnut, *Obstetric Anesthesia*, pp. 126–27.

36. Ibid., p. 141.

37. T. K. Abboud et al., "Maternal, Fetal, and Neonatal Responses after Epidural Anesthesia with Bupivacaine, 2-Chloroprocaine, or Lidocaine," *Anesthesia and Analgesia* 61, no. 8 (1982): 638–44.

38. Abboud et al., "Comparison of the Effects."

39. Reynolds et al., "Analgesia in Labour."

Glossary

———————◆———————

*Y*OU WILL WANT TO refer to the text for a more complete explanation of terms.

Anesthesia Medically induced loss of sensation (pain) with or without loss of consciousness. *See also types of anesthesia:* local, regional, spinal, epidural, and general.

Anesthesiologist A medical doctor who specializes in anesthesia. In the United States, an anesthesiologist completes medical school or osteopathic medical school and then trains for an additional four years in medicine and anesthesia.

Anesthetist In the United States, "anesthetist" usually refers to a nurse-anesthetist. *See also* CRNA.

Attending Also called "attending physician." A medical doctor who has completed his or her specialty training as a resident. *Compare to* intern and resident.

Birth canal A passageway, formed by the cervix and vagina, for the baby during birth.

Bolus *See* epidural bolus.

Catheter A flexible, often plastic, tube through which fluids can be withdrawn or medications injected.

Cervix The lower section of the uterus that dilates during labor to form a passageway for the baby during birth.

Cesarean section (C-section) The surgical procedure in the lower abdomen to deliver (remove) the baby from the uterus (womb).

Combined spinal epidural (CSE, walking epidural) The loss of sensation (pain) to a region of the body by injection of medication into both the epidural space and the fluid surrounding the spinal cord. A CSE is one type of regional anesthesia.

Contraction *See* uterine contraction.

CRNA Certified registered nurse-anesthetist.

CSE *See* combined spinal epidural.

C-section *See* Cesarean section.

Epidural *See* epidural anesthesia.

Epidural anesthesia The loss of sensation (pain) to a region of the body by injection of medication into the epidural space. Epidural anesthesia is one type of regional anesthesia.

Epidural bolus (bolus, top up) An additional dose of epidural medication that expands the volume of medication within the epidural space. An epidural bolus is usually stronger in concentration than the medication in the epidural infusion.

Epidural catheter An extremely thin, flexible, plastic tube that sits in the epidural space. It permits the injection of medications into the epidural space.

Epidural infusion Medication infused via a mechanical device through an epidural catheter and into the epidural space. An epidural infusion is used to maintain the epidural anesthesia throughout labor.

Epidural space The space just outside both the spinal cord and the spinal cord's surrounding fluid. Nerves emanating from the spinal cord first pass through the epidural space before heading out to different parts of the body.

Fetal heart rate (FHR) The baby's heart rate monitored during labor. The changes in FHR as they correspond to uterine contractions are a measure of the baby's well-being.

General anesthesia The loss of sensation (pain) *with* the loss of consciousness. General anesthesia can be administered by injection of medications into a vein or by inhalation of medications.

Intern A medical doctor in his or her first year of specialty training after medical school. *Compare to* attending and resident.

Intravenous (IV) A small catheter inserted into a vein to permit fluid and medications to be administered quickly and easily into the bloodstream. The catheter is usually connected to tubing and a bag of sterile fluid.

IV *See* intravenous.

L&D *See* labor and delivery.

Labor A process that involves uterine contractions, dilation of the cervix, and the passage of the baby from the uterus through the birth canal.

Labor and delivery Labor and the birth of a baby.

Labor and delivery unit The place in the hospital where babies are born. Also called L&D, L&D unit, birthing unit, birthing ward, obstetric unit, or obstetric ward.

Labor pain Pain experienced from labor.

Local anesthesia The loss of sensation (pain) by the direct injection of medication into and around the area causing pain.

Local anesthetic Medication that temporarily blocks signals that travel along nerves. Local anesthetics are used in local and regional anesthesia, including epidural and spinal anesthesia.

Maternal fever A rise in body temperature above normal in an expectant mother.

Narcotic Medications that interact with special receptors in the spinal cord and brain. Narcotics have multiple effects, including blunting the sensation of pain.

Nerve A specialized group of cells that form a "living wire" to carry information to and from the brain.

Nurse-anesthetist *See* CNRA.

OB *See* obstetrics.

OB doctor *See* obstetrician.

OB-GYN Refers to the medical field of obstetrics and gynecology.

OB nurse A nurse specializing in the care of pregnant women.

Obstetrician A doctor specializing in the care of pregnant women.

Obstetrics The medical field specializing in pregnancy and childbirth.

Operating room (OR) A specialized room in the hospital where surgery is performed.

OR *See* operating room.

Pain signal A biochemical message initiated from a painful stimulus conducted along a nerve to the brain.

Patient-controlled analgesia (PCA) An IV narcotic infusion connected to a device. The device allows the expectant mother to decide when and how often she receives extra IV narcotic medication (with built-in safety parameters).

Patient-controlled epidural analgesia (PCEA) An epidural infusion connected to a device. The device allows the expectant mother to decide when and how often she receives extra epidural medication (with built-in safety parameters).

PCA *See* patient-controlled anesthesia.

PCEA *See* patient-controlled epidural anesthesia.

Postdural puncture headache *See* spinal headache.

Regional anesthesia The loss of sensation (pain) by the injection of medication near nerves that are conducting pain signals from a body part to the brain. Both epidural and spinal anesthesia are types of regional anesthesia.

Resident A medical doctor in his or her second or greater year of specialty training after medical school. The specialty training may be in obstetrics and gynecology, anesthesiology, pediatrics, etc. *Compare to* attending and intern.

Spinal *See* spinal anesthesia.

Spinal anesthesia The loss of sensation (pain) to a region of the body by injection of medication into the fluid surrounding the spinal cord. Spinal anesthesia is one type of regional anesthesia.

Spinal column (spine) The column of bones forming the central structural support of the body. The spine also forms an internal channel in which the spinal cord descends from the brain.

Spinal cord The bundle of nerves extending from the brain down through the spine. Nerves branch off the spinal cord to innervate the body.

Spinal headache (postdural puncture headache) A headache due to a spinal or an epidural.

Spine *See* spinal column.

Teaching hospital A hospital affiliated with a medical school and/or residency training program(s) where students and doctors learn from experienced physicians.

Test dose A small amount of medication initially injected through an epidural catheter to confirm its placement within the epidural space.

Top up *See* epidural bolus.

Uterine contraction The rhythmic muscular squeezing of the uterus during labor.

Uterus The organ in an expectant mother where her baby lives and grows until childbirth.

Uterus-cervix area The uterus and cervix.

Vaginal-rectal area The vagina, rectum, and adjacent area.

Walking epidural *See* combined spinal epidural.

Index

acid-base status of newborns, 108

acupuncture, 99

addiction to pain medication, risk of, 94–95

allergic reactions, 63

anesthesia: conditions affecting, 64–71; for C-section, 79; effects on baby, 88–89, 101–8; general, 2, 88–90, 105; local, 21; options for, 3–4, 72–77, 79–83, 87, 96–99; rare complications of, 59–63; recovering from effects of, 91–93; regional, 2, 72–76, 79, 101; uncommon complications of, 50–58. *See also* safety of anesthesia; spinal anesthetic

anesthesiologist: choice of, 9; communication style of, 22, 29, 44–45; health insurance and, 11; requesting early visit with, 17–18, 67, 68, 70–71

antacid, liquid, 81

APGAR score, 48, 106

auditory changes, 56, 57

baby: comfort of, 13; holding after C-section, 86; sight of after C-section, 85

baby, effects on: acid-base status, 108; APGAR score, 106; dose of medication, 38–39; general anesthesia, 88–89; IV pain medication, 98; neurobehavioral testing, 107; regional anesthesia (epidurals and spinals), 48, 79, 101–8

back problems: bulging discs, 65–67; after delivery, 50–52; before pregnancy and delivery, 65–68

back surgery, 68

bleeding abnormalities, 61, 69–70

blood: clotting ability of, 61, 69–71; flow of, to uterus and placenta, 48, 103–4

blood patch, epidural, 56–57

blood pressure: decrease in, 46–48; dose of medication and, 38–39; after epidural, 16

blood tests: for blood abnormalities, 70, 71; before epidural, 18; umbilical cord, 48

blood thinners, 61, 69, 70

boluses, 38–39, 40, 76–77

breech position, 78

bulging discs, 65–67

bupivicaine, 31, 49

"-caine" medications, 1–2, 31, 49

"call," taking, 10

catheter, epidural: description of, 7; location of, 26, 36, 37, 39; medicine supplied through, 28–29, 30–31, 38–39, 76–78, 83; placement of, 25–27, 50; removal of, 91; replacement of, 42–43; taping of, 22, 27, 42